D1544034

COUPLE THERAPY FOR INFERTILITY

THE GUILFORD FAMILY THERAPY SERIES

Michael P. Nichols, Series Editor

Recent Volumes

Couple Therapy for Infertility
Ronny Diamond, David Kezur, Mimi Meyers,
Constance N. Scharf, and Margot Weinshel

Short-Term Couple Therapy
James M. Donovan, Editor

Treating the Tough Adolescent: A Family-Based,
Step-by-Step Guide
Scott P. Sells

Strengthening Family Resilience
Froma Walsh

The Adolescent in Family Therapy: Breaking the Cycle
of Conflict and Control
Joseph A. Micucci

Working with Families of the Poor
Patricia Minuchin, Jorge Colapinto, and Salvador Minuchin

Latino Families in Therapy: A Guide to Multicultural Practice
Celia Jaes Falicov

Essential Skills in Family Therapy: From the First Interview
to Termination
JoEllen Patterson, Lee Williams, Claudia Grauf-Grounds,
and Larry Chamow

Case Studies in Couple and Family Therapy:
Systemic and Cognitive Perspectives
Frank M. Dattilio, Editor

COUPLE THERAPY FOR INFERTILITY

Ronny Diamond
David Kezur
Mimi Meyers
Constance N. Scharf
Margot Weinshel

THE GUILFORD PRESS
NEW YORK   LONDON

© 1999 The Guilford Press
A Division of Guilford Publications, Inc.
72 Spring Street, New York, NY 10012
http://www.guilford.com

Printed in the United States of America

This book is printed on acid-free paper.

Last digit is print number: 9 8 7 6 5 4 3 2 1

Library of Congress Cataloging-in-Publication Data

Couple therapy for infertility / Ronny Diamond . . . [et al.].
    p. cm.—(The Guilford family therapy series)
  Includes bibliographical references and index.
  ISBN 1-57230-511-8
  1. Infertility—Psychological aspects. 2. Infertility—Patients—
Counseling of. 3. Marital psychotherapy. I. Diamond, Ronny.
II. Series.
RC889.C68 1999
616.6′9206—dc21   99-16283
                                                   CIP

*To the couples whose struggles, anguish, sorrow,
and joy made this work possible.*

ABOUT THE AUTHORS

Ronny Diamond, MSW, is a member of the Infertility Project at the Ackerman Institute for the Family. She is Director of Post Adoption Services at Spence-Chapin Services to Families and Children and has a private practice in New York City.

David Kezur, MSW, is on the teaching faculty of the Ackerman Institute for the Family and is also a member of Ackerman's Infertility Project. He has a private practice in New York City.

Mimi Meyers, MSW, is on the teaching faculty of the Ackerman Institute for the Family, and is also a member of Ackerman's Infertility Project. She has a private practice in Manhattan and Brooklyn, New York.

Constance N. Scharf, MSW, is on the teaching faculty of the Ackerman Institute for the Family, where she serves as the Dean of Students and is also a member of Ackerman's Infertility Project. She is an adjunct teaching assistant in the Department of Psychiatry at the Mount Sinai Hospital and has a private practice in New York City.

Margot Weinshel, MSW, RN, is on the teaching faculty of the Ackerman Institute for the Family and is a member of Ackerman's Infertility Project. She is a Family Therapy Supervisor, Family Studies Program, New York University Child Studies Center, and coauthor of *Surviving an Eating Disorder*. She has a private practice in New York City.

ACKNOWLEDGMENTS

❧

We are grateful to the Ackerman Institute for the Family for its support and nurturance of our work, for its climate of intellectual discovery, and for its spirit of clinical innovation. With special thanks to Peter Steinglass, MD, the Institute's Director, whose support and guidance made our project and this text possible.

We thank Seymour Weingarten, who, with reassuring confidence in our work, helped keep us on track. Michael Nichols, PhD, a superb editor, gave us excellent feedback. Our thanks to Kimberley Windbiel for organizing our manuscript, and for her certainty that there would be a day—within our lifetimes—on which the book would be published. Kitty Moore continued the process and helped to move it forward.

We appreciate our colleagues' support at the Ackerman Institute for the Family: Virginia Goldner, PhD, who encouraged us to write our book; Arthur Maslow, MSW, whose NIFTY funds provided the seed money for our initial work; Marcia Sheinberg, MSW, Director of Training and Clinical Services, who has supported our work and encouraged our efforts to bring our ideas to a larger clinical audience; Peggy Penn, MSW, who, as teacher, colleague, and friend, contributed to making each of us better thinkers, clinicians, and humanitarians; Evan Imber-Black, PhD, for sharing her ideas on donor disclosure; Peter Fraenkel, PhD, Director of Research, who was a valuable research consultant; Climeen Wikoff, MFA, Ackerman's talented and unruffled Video Coordinator; and the Institute's skilled and hard-working support staff—Miranda Aaron, MSW; Kenya Aska, Melanie, Benvenue, Susan

Delaney, Erlyne Evans, Leslye Lynford, Brian McCullough, and Suna O'Neill.

We give thanks to the many couples who were willing to share their lives and struggles with us and our readers. And, lastly, we are grateful to our families who were, for the most part, able to endure our seemingly interminable writing retreats, and who provided support (sometimes conditional) and love (always unconditional): (R. D.) Tom Levin, Jason Samuels, and Natasha Page-Levin; (D. K.) JoEllen Fisherkeller; (M. M.) Gary Mangus, Joan, and Greg Meyers; (C. N. S.) Robert, Jeremiah, and Melissa Scharf; (M. W.) Robert, Rebecca, Josh, and Stephanie Bazell.

CONTENTS

INTRODUCTION

From early in childhood, most people expect to grow up, get married, and have children. When infertility strikes, it usually takes couples by surprise. Stunned and incredulous, they turn to the medical arena where they begin a process that is likely to leave them emotionally exhausted and physically invaded. Feeling out of control; misunderstood by friends, family, and society; and suffering a loss of confidence in themselves and each other, partners are likely to find that infertility presents a grave challenge to their sense of identity as individuals and as a couple.

Until recently, infertility was not acknowledged as a major life crisis. Now, despite this increased awareness, misconceptions persist, both about the causes of infertility and the degree of its impact. Couple and family therapists are only beginning to recognize the distress caused by the ordeal of infertility and the painful legacies it leaves in its wake.

The Infertility Project was organized at the Ackerman Institute for the Family in 1991 to address the lack of understanding about the effects of infertility on couples. As senior faculty members, we have benefited from the Institute's support and encouragement to investigate specific problems and generate innovative treatment models for work with particular populations. Our group was drawn together by our mutual interest in couple therapy and by our awareness that infertility represented a significant but poorly understood therapeutic challenge. We were also struck by the fact that nearly all of the literature we encountered focused on the trauma of infertility as an individual problem. We decided to work with couples experiencing infertility because we believe that in spite of the fact that a woman's body is the site of the treatment, both partners feel infertility's effects, and therefore the couple relationship can be affected. In addition, one of us had had a first-hand encounter with infertility: After being told in her late 20s that she was infertile, she entered the medical arena in her late 30s and finally gave birth to a child through *in vitro* fertilization.

We began by recruiting couples who were struggling with infertility. In the Institute's one-way mirrored interview rooms, individual couples and their treating clinician met while the team observed the sessions from behind the mirror and developed ideas. In the beginning, we focused on learning as much as possible about couples' experiences by inviting them to "tell us their story." Many couples presented with an initial wariness; feeling marginalized and misunderstood by friends, family, and society, they often expected similar reactions from us. In fact, during our initial meetings with couples they often told us how gratifying it was to know that the Project existed. Couples felt that the Ackerman Institute and the prestige it commanded in the field of family therapy lent legitimacy to the difficulty of their plight.

As we gained understanding of how couples were experiencing their infertility, we applied many techniques used in standard systemic couple therapy, which we described in a paper published in *Family Process* (Meyers et al., 1995b). These include the following:

> (1) exploring particular problems that couples presented, and how each partner experienced them; (2) tracking the interactional patterns of the couple (including communication patterns); (3) mapping the couple's relationships with family and other networks (including the medical systems); (4) unearthing the paradigms, beliefs, and legacies that colored each partner's experiences of all of the above; and (5) offering couples opportunities to transform problematic assumptions and interactional patterns.

In time, as we began to fine-tune our treatment and develop specific protocols for working with couples struggling with infertility, we noticed that there appeared to be a pattern to the progression of their experience. What emerged were identifiable phases to the infertility ordeal. This led us to develop the model presented in this book, which has been helpful to us in diagnosing a couple's phase-specific experiences and finding appropriate interventions.

Our culture, like most, has placed great value on having and parenting children; in fact, we are often described as a child-centered society. Although most of the couples with whom we work plan to have children, there are others who prefer to live their lives without children. These couples' decisions may reflect their ethical orientation, namely that the world's burgeoning population exceeds our planet's shrinking resources; others prefer to put their life efforts into careers and other interests. Sometimes the decision not to have children is a combination of both.

As clinicians, we are often faced with the question of how to refer to couples without children. It is a difficult decision because each of the two conventional terms, "childless" and "childfree," has very different implications, and each implies a particular perspective on the matter. The "-less" in "childless" denotes the absence of something—a deficiency. Couples struggling with infertility are generally unhappy with this label because it carries a sense of the tragic; throughout the ages, "childlessness" has been regarded as a misfortune. However, the term "childfree," while appearing to be a neutral description, implies a preferred state of being. Although childfree may be an accurate self-definition for couples who choose to live their lives without children, it is less suitable for couples actively struggling with infertility who do not have any choice in this matter. In order to resolve this linguistic dilemma, we refer to these couples as "without children," unless we are describing a particular couple who has elected to be childfree.

This leads to another label that gives us pause, namely, "infertile." Because the experience of infertility brings with it associations of deviance and defect, and because it is an experience mired in failure, it is common for one or both partners to feel that they are personal failures and inherently defective. A label such as "infertile" is likely to reinforce a negative view of the self that supersedes all other descriptions. For example, one woman said, "Although I am a store manager, a Democrat, a Protestant, a daughter, a wife, an aunt, and lots of other things, I see myself as infertile more than anything else." Therefore, we prefer to use the noun "infertility," as this allows people to separate themselves from their condition. We also use the term "struggling with infertility," which places couples in an active position with a sense of agency.

Using this kind of semantic tool in practice, we might say, "How long have the two of you been struggling with infertility?" rather than saying, "How long have you been infertile?" Although the phrase "struggling with infertility" is more cumbersome than "infertile," we hope that the reader/clinician will become accustomed to thinking about and referring to couples in this semantic frame, and thereby feel more comfortable using it in his or her therapy sessions.

Infertility strikes all kinds of couples—married, unmarried, heterosexual, and gay. However, the couples with whom we worked were predominantly married heterosexuals. Therefore, in regard to language used in this book, when specifically discussing the treatment group we may refer to husbands, wives, and marriage.

As we began to share our work with other therapists, they often expressed that they felt at a loss about how to proceed effectively with these couples. They were not clear about the unique issues about infertility, and tended to take a problem-solving stance without considering the significance of a couple's beliefs about parenting and children, identity issues associated with masculinity and femininity, and the impact on the couple relationship. Too often the woman became the client, and the couple dynamics were overlooked.

This book is structured in the following way: Chapter 1 introduces the demographics and psychology of infertility, along with our phase-specific model. Chapter 2 provides an overview of our therapeutic approach.

Chapters 3–14 describe the phase model of infertility that we have observed: Dawning, Mobilization, Immersion, Resolution, and Legacy. For each phase there are two chapters, in which we discuss the Couple Issues and then the Therapeutic Approach that can be employed during the particular phase. In the latter part of the Immersion phase, couples may face the decision of whether or not to use donor gametes (i.e., sperm or eggs). As this complex topic is distinct from the issues encountered earlier in the Immersion phase, we have divided this phase into two sections, Early and Middle Immersion and Late Immersion. In Chapter 15, we conclude briefly with future directions for research and suggest how professionals in the fields of mental health and medicine can help couples to cope with infertility.

During the years of the Infertility Project, we have become aware that infertility is a "make or break" (Rolland, 1994) experience. We have been gratified that many of the couples in the Project reported improvements in their ability to make informed medical decisions, in their marital satisfaction, and in their preparation for parenthood or for a life without children. In a series of follow-up interviews, we have found these changes to be lasting.

> "The Ackerman therapy has been very valuable. I used to think this marriage wasn't going to last, but now our relationship is very solid. I've come to realize this is really about our marriage. It's not about the infertility anymore. We are two of the lucky ones. We've been able to use the infertility to unite us rather than drive us apart."

1

&

THE ISSUES AND PHASES
OF INFERTILITY

From time immemorial, fertility has been a primal concern for human society. From the Venus of Willendorf, the plump fertility goddess of prehistoric Europe, through the Biblical injunction to "be fruitful and multiply," fecundity has been highly prized, ensuring the survival of the species and of the particular tribe or nation. Children provide existential meaning, identity, and status; they grant parents the traditional means of participating in the continuity of a family, a culture, and the human race (Meyers et al., 1995b). Conversely, the inability to bear children has been pitied and feared. The language of infertility—barren, unfruitful, fallow, impotent—carries powerful associations, and many primitive religious activities focused on preventing it. The infertile have been scorned or shunned, and infertility has often had negative consequences ranging from grounds for annulment, as in the case of Anne of Cleves, Henry VIII's fourth wife, to, during the Inquisition, proof of consorting with the Devil.

In modern times, attitudes have changed in the face of overpopulation, effective birth control, and educated populations (particularly of women). Witness, for example, China's prohibition against having more than one child and the increased rates of voluntary sterilization in India. In Western culture, the 1950s' focus on family was supplanted by a concentration on women's career development during the 1960s and 1970s, spurred in part by the availability of birth control pills and the IUD.

However, fertility is still highly prized. Most North American cou-

5

ples plan to have children when they get married (Mathews, 1991), and people often choose a mate based partly on expectations of what he or she will be like as a parent. After marriage, "preparation for the anticipated children can be highly structured" (Meyers et al., 1995b). In addition, using contraception reinforces couples' supposition that they are fertile.

Infertility is defined as the inability either to achieve a pregnancy after a year of regular sexual relations without the use of contraception or to carry a pregnancy to live birth (Merck Manual, 1992). *Primary infertility* occurs in couples who have never had a child, and *secondary infertility* refers to those who experience the inability either to conceive or to achieve a live birth after previously bearing one or more children. Infertility can be treated medically, and 80% of infertile couples will conceive within 4–5 years of diagnosis. However, birth rates for those who never receive medical treatment are only 6% lower than for those who enter the medical arena (Jones & Toner, 1993).

Those who encounter difficulty conceiving face a variety of myths about infertility. One of the most prevalent is that all the couple has to do is "just relax and you'll get pregnant." However, this echoes the attitudes of the 1950s and 1960s, when only 30–40% of infertility could be diagnosed (Eisner, 1963), and infertility was often attributed to psychological dysfunctions such as women's hostility toward their mothers or partners, aggressive imitation of the male, and ambivalence toward motherhood (Benedek, 1952). Now, however, diagnostic procedures offer physiological explanations for 90% of infertility cases (Meyers et al., 1995a). Although infertility is often considered a women's problem because the woman's body is the site of most treatments, male and female factors both contribute, with male factors accounting for 40% of infertility; female factors, 40%; interactive factors between men and women, 10%; whereas 10% remain unexplained or *idiopathic* (Marrs, 1997).

With regard to stress affecting fertility, Domar, Seibel, and Benson (1990) have studied the use of relaxation techniques to help infertile women cope with the stresses of infertility treatments. A surprisingly high percentage of patients achieved pregnancy after participating in the program. However, there is a distinct possibility that the successes may have occurred with cases of unexplained infertility (only 10% of cases), rather than identifiable medical conditions such as endometriosis (when the endometrial tissue grows outside the uterus) or azoospermia (no sperm). Although this research into the mind/body connection certainly holds interest for the future, it is important not to "blame the victim" by reverting to the suggestion that the individual's psychological state is the cause of infertility.

A second myth is associated with the fact that within the last decade, infertility has received increasing media coverage, which often emphasizes the most sensational aspects of treatment and profiles couples who elect the most radical procedures. Because of this increased attention, it would seem that the condition is becoming an epidemic. In fact, infertility is not affecting a greater *proportion* of couples. The absolute number of infertile people has grown (approximately 10 million individuals; Berger, Goldstein, & Fuerst, 1995) in part because the baby boom generation is so large, but the percentage has remained at about 10% of married couples for the past 25 years (Marrs, 1997). The only segment of the population to have a proportional increase in infertility is young women aged 20–24, among whom infertility grew from 4% in 1965 to 11% in 1982. This change is attributed to a rise in sexually transmitted diseases (STDs), which can affect fertility. In addition, contrary to popular misconception, rather than being merely a "yuppie malady" (Meyers et al., 1995a) spawned by baby boomers delaying family to concentrate on career, infertility strikes hardest among poor people of color with little formal education (U.S. Office of Technology Assessment, 1988).

However, another reason for the growing number of infertile couples is, in fact, that more couples are delaying childbearing. This has occurred for a number of reasons including women's desires to have careers and couples' wishes to achieve a certain level of financial stability before they start their families. Since the mid-1960s, the proportion of married women under 30 delaying childbearing has jumped from 12% to 25%, and women over 30 accounted for 1 out of 3 U.S. births in 1992 (Berger et al., 1995). Because fertility declines over time, this means that couples have fewer years to achieve a pregnancy. Although men's fertility may decrease with age for a variety of reasons including alcohol consumption, smoking, STDs, or a worsening of a varicocele (a varicose vein in the testicle), as reproductive technology stands now, women's decrease in fertility is biologically inevitable. Women's infertility rates increase with age: Approximately 10% of women age 15–30, 14% of women age 30–34, and 25% of women 35 and older experience infertility problems. The decline is rapid after age 35, with infertility rising to 30% by age 37, 45% by age 40, and 70% by age 43 (Mosher & Pratt, 1990).

Another current perception about infertility holds that women have brought it on themselves by deserting their traditional roles in society; women who aspire to having both careers and families are seen as spoiled and selfish. This third myth ignores the sociobiological forces that compel couples to delay childbearing. Although men who want to be more active fathers may want to ensure that their careers are solid and that they have the financial resources to allow them to spend time with their children, the dilemma facing today's couples is that many women must gamble on how long they can stay on a career ladder without forfeiting their fertility. They worry that if they leave the workplace too soon, they will not only jeopardize their careers, but may also compromise their family's financial security and hence their children's well-being. In postponing pregnancy, Judy faced a common dilemma:

> "I wanted to wait until I was established enough in my career to leave and then get a job that would allow me to keep some status—enough for me to take off if my kid got sick, or if I had to visit his school, or just stay home and make cookies. I didn't want to worry that my commitment to my work would be questioned. . . . There's a woman at work who got pregnant when she was in a lower level of management; she came back to the same job and hasn't moved since. Nobody takes her seriously. . . . If I wasn't worried about that, we would've had kids several years ago. So, now that I earned enough respect to go back after having a kid and hang onto my reputation, what does the doctor say? My biological equipment's too old."

Many women have witnessed their own mothers' lives and regard them as cautionary tales of women sacrificing their personal development in order to raise children. Carolyn, an interior decorator, described her reasoning:

> "I worried that I would be like my mother; she was an accomplished cellist who could never go back to it once us kids came along. She was a sad women, full of regrets, a little envious of me, I think; there's a gulf between us. . . . I want to be a fuller person for any daughter I would have. I want my child to respect my life. . . . But . . . in trying to become . . . a good role model, I've jeopardized having a child to be a good mother to!"

In addition, some couples delay having children because of their ambivalence about children or the relationship, whereas others may choose to delay childbearing until they have reached a certain level of emotional and relational maturity. Although this choice may be related to their wish to develop their careers, the motivation is also to develop as individuals, to enjoy the pleasures of life without children, and to enhance their relationship with each other. As a result, there may be a gap between a couple's sense of psychological readiness for children and their biological fitness for reproduction.

One consequence of waiting is the increased risk of infertility. Paradoxically, a second consequence can mitigate the first: Couples who have had an opportunity to develop full lives without children, who have alternative means of satisfying their desire to have creative lives and rich connections to friends, may be better able to cope with the infertility and/or resolving the loss of a genetically related child (Ireland, 1993). Yet, in spite of the mitigating effects of delaying childbirth, infertility remains a distressing development for most couples.

A fourth myth holds that once a couple has had children, they should have little difficulty achieving pregnancy in the future. However, secondary infertility—occurring in couples or individuals who have had at least one live birth, but then have trouble having another child— occurs with approximately 10% of parents. Surprisingly, secondary infertility is estimated to account for 50–70% of infertility (Simons, 1995). However, this phenomenon is not widely recognized. Secondary infertility may be more dismaying to couples than primary infertility because it is so unexpected. In addition, secondary infertility often garners less sympathy and understanding than primary infertility: Because the couple already has at least one child, family and friends cannot understand their distress over being unable to have another. However, many couples feel a deep sense of loss about not being able to achieve their desired family size or to provide their child with siblings. Social expectations about family composition can also contribute to couples' discomfort, as in the following example from a religious couple:

> Although Hannah already had three children, she was devastated by the diagnosis of secondary infertility. In her orthodox Jewish community where having many children is highly prized, Hannah felt that her identity as a woman was highly compromised by the diagnosis.

COUPLE ISSUES

Researchers have confirmed that couples who desire but cannot have biological children are often profoundly distressed. Researchers have examined the effects of infertility on individuals from a variety of perspectives. Infertility can be been viewed as a life crisis (Burns, 1990; Kedem, Mikulincer, Nathanson, & Bartov, 1990), an identity crisis (Bassin, 1989; Greil, 1991; Hendricks, 1985), a chronic illness (Sandelowski, 1993), a trauma (Humphrey, 1986), a cause of grief and mourning (Menning, 1988; Myers, 1990), and an existential experience, as well as any combination of these.

The value of comparing infertility to trauma has significant limits in that there is variation from couple to couple. Individuals respond differently to the diagnosis and to treatments: Some can contain their anguish while awaiting more information, others seem traumatized by the mere suggestion of some subfertile condition. Still others greet the diagnosis with relative equanimity, but are traumatized by miscarriages; and another group does not experience the trauma in reaction to a distinct event, but rather at an unspecific time when an identity dominated by infertility takes hold. The length of time dealing with infertility can also affect the way it is experienced. Therefore, depending on the particular person, either a chronic illness or a crisis template may be the most appropriate way to understand the experience.

As the physiological causes of infertility were discovered, research began to focus on the psychological *impact* rather than the psychological *causes* of infertility (Seibel & Taymor, 1982). Because most research is conducted with couples who have sought medical treatment or those who constitute only one segment of the infertile population, it is not clear whether the findings indicate a skewed distress reaction. Nonetheless, several common psychological reactions to the infertility experience have been noted by researchers.

The Crisis and Trauma of Infertility

For many, infertility poses a challenge to their most deeply held beliefs about themselves and the world around them. In terms of stressful life experiences, infertility is often rated as high as the death of a child or a spouse (Kedem et al., 1990). This blow to their identity hits many as a crisis (Humphrey, 1986), with women who struggle with infertility being more likely than their fertile counterparts to experience higher levels of anxiety, tension, guilt, anger, and depression (O'Moore, O'Moore, Harrison, & Carruthers, 1983).

Loss and Mourning

Individuals who are struggling with infertility experience many losses. First and foremost, there is the loss of having a genetically related child and the associated life experiences including pregnancy, carrying forth one's family lineage, creating a child with one's partner, and so forth (Clamar, 1980). Added to these are losses of life goals, status, prestige, and self-confidence (Burns, 1990; Mahlstedt, 1985). Mourning these losses is an essential aspect of resolving infertility (Menning, 1988; Myers, 1990). However, couples struggling with infertility often simultaneously hold two conflicting thoughts about the future. Compared to someone facing a death, when the mourner must accept the irrefutable loss of the loved one, these couples may be mourning the loss of future children while at the same time participating in treatments that encourage them to feel hopeful about having a baby. Because there is little middle ground where one can adapt to this ambiguous future, oscillations of hope and despair are common.

Impact on the Couple Relationship

Infertility presents a severe challenge to a couple's relationship (Andrews, Abbey, & Halman, 1992; Berg & Wilson, 1991; Burns, 1990; Daniluk, 1988; Hirsch & Hirsch, 1989; Morse & Dennerstein, 1985; Shaw, Johnston, & Shaw, 1988), with partners encountering many difficulties including problems with communication, sexual functioning, and decision making. Once they have entered the medical arena and are undergoing diagnostic evaluations and procedures, many couples report conflict, disagreements over medical treatments, failure of empathy, and differential investments in the process. Particular areas of difficulty include keeping secrets and protecting each other from negative thoughts and feelings, being "out of synch" in terms of emotional and physical investment in the process, gender differences in terms of degree of impact and coping, and disturbances in the sexual relationship.

Secrecy and Protection

As couples begin to feel guilt and resentment about infertility, they may become reluctant to discuss these thoughts and feelings with their partners. Motivated by a desire to protect the other from feelings of shame or defect, and wanting to conceal their own depression, anger, hurt, and fantasies of flight, partners shut down communication, cutting off an avenue of support and consolation at a time when it is sorely needed.

Out of Synch

Each partner may move through the feelings and thoughts about infertility at a different pace. Thus, as each progresses on his or her own timetable, they may find that they are out of synch with each other in terms of many of the emotional processes and the important decisions that infertility engenders, for example, readiness to undertake a certain medical procedure, the need to mourn the losses of infertility, or how much financial investment to make in treatment. If these discrepancies are not addressed, they can lead to problems for the couple during the ordeal and in its aftermath.

Gender Differences

Men and women often use different coping and communication styles. As in many other areas of life, this may also hold true during the ordeal of infertility. Failure to recognize and address these issues can lead to misunderstanding and conflict in the couple's relationship.

Sexual Relationship

Infertility often has a damaging impact on a couple's sexual relationship. When couples first attempt to conceive, freedom from having to use contraception may feel liberating. But, as time goes by with no pregnancy, love making often becomes associated with fear and failure, and sexual relations can begin to turn sour. In addition, the necessity of scheduling sexual intercourse to coincide with times of prime fertility leads to a loss of spontaneity, such that sex can feel mechanical and passionless (Berg & Wilson, 1991).

The Infertile Identity

Unable to proceed to the childrearing stage in life, couples struggling with infertility often feel they are outside the mainstream, stigmatized as different and, essentially, defective. As time goes on, with pregnancy remaining elusive, an *infertile identity* can take root. Infertility becomes a "social disability" (Menning, 1988), and couples may be regarded as deviant and unnatural in a child-centered society that is ignorant of the impact of infertility (Sandelowski, 1993).

Gender Differences

The infertile identity produces its own set of problematic gender differences in that although both men and women take on the infertile identity, women experience significantly more distress (Freeman, Boxer, Rickels, Tureck, & Mastrioanni, 1985). However, over time, gender differences tend to diminish (Berg & Wilson, 1991).

The Couple and the Support System

As couples struggle with infertility, ruptures may occur in their relations with their family and friends. In response to questions about their plans to start a family, couples may respond by either revealing their struggle or choosing not to discuss it. There are pitfalls to each strategy. If they choose to discuss their infertility, couples may face more embarrassing questions and useless, unsolicited advice such as "just relax." If they remain silent, they risk isolating themselves and having few allies to support them in their distress.

Couples may find that others regard infertility treatment as an unwarranted self-indulgence. Unlike fertile couples, whose choice to procreate is not questioned, couples who elect to use assisted reproductive technology (ART) such as *in vitro* fertilization or donor procedures (see the Appendix) in order to have genetically related children are often called upon to defend their choices (Bartholet, 1993). RESOLVE, a national self-help organization, was founded to counter the sense of isolation and marginalization that these couples experience.

In addition, social activities that once were enjoyable, such as child-centered family parties, may now be so painful and upsetting that couples prefer to avoid them. Friends and family may respond with hurt or criticism, or they may be so overly solicitous that couples feel as though they are regarded as pathetic.

The Couple and the Medical System

As couples enter the infertility medical system, a whole new set of intense relationships develops with doctors, nurses, lab technicians, and so forth (Burns, 1990; McDaniel, Hepworth, & Doherty, 1992). Hoping that the doctor will provide them with a child and fearing that he or she will not, couples often compromise their autonomy in an effort to be "good patients" in order to ensure that they get the best treatment (Mahlstedt, 1985). Couples also face a daunting array of medical procedures to treat infertility. Not only will they need to make difficult decisions, but the treatments themselves are time consuming and physically and emotionally stressful.

The challenges infertility poses to the couple relationship are many. The stresses can unearth old conflicts and deeply ingrained family-of-origin patterns. Those who are able to work through the ordeal together often find that it strengthens their sense of intimacy and commitment to the relationship (Greil, 1991).

THE PHASES OF INFERTILITY

After working with couples in the Infertility Project, we began to notice that, in general, the ordeal has a trajectory, and that there are five distinct phases: *Dawning, Mobilization, Immersion, Resolution*, and *Legacy*. Although the transitions from one phase to another are often subtle, each has distinctive features. Particular issues cluster in each phase, and by understanding the trajectory of couples' distress, the therapist is better able to gauge their level of entrenchment, that is, the extent to which the negative effects of infertility have created significant disruption in the partners' interactional patterns. In addition, it is helpful for the clinician to know that certain issues will be more pertinent at different times in the progression; for example, although the theme of loss may be touched upon briefly in the Mobilization phase, it becomes of paramount importance in Resolution. Thus, these phases can give the clinician a framework in which to view couples' distress, and they can also be used to guide couples as they navigate the stormy waters of infertility.

We should note, however, that as with any phase model of human behavior, this set of stages should be viewed as a fluid, and often recursive process, rather than as a linear, progressive structure. Thus, we use the phases not so much to move couples through their crises, but rather to monitor their progress and offer appropriate assistance.

• During the Dawning phase, couples become increasingly aware that they may have a problem conceiving. This concern grows with each month's failure to conceive until, by the end of the phase, this fear becomes strong enough that the couple seeks a medical consultation.

• Mobilization marks the first step into the medical arena as couples begin diagnostic testing. Although they may be concerned about the possibility of infertility, a definitive diagnosis is likely to cause shock and disbelief, particularly in cases of secondary infertility. Problems may begin to emerge in the relationship as couples face the first loss of infertility: a "normal," problem-free conception.

• Immersion is the most complex and demanding phase. As couples undergo more testing and medical treatments, they remain in a liminal, "not yet pregnant" state (Greil, 1991), a limbo from which they cannot move ahead into the next stage of the life cycle, that is, parenting. Instead, they are tossed endlessly back and forth between hope that they will have a child and despair at the thought that they may not. Battered by the duress of medical procedures, loss of privacy and control of the body, and anticipatory grief at the possibility of being childless (Sandelowski, 1993), this is often a time of turmoil in a couple's relationship. Late in Immersion, if they have been unable to conceive a child, couples may be offered the option of using donor gametes (sperm or eggs[1]). Although this is often treated as simply another rung on the treatment ladder, adding another person's gametes to the family equation produces

---

[1]Although ovum/ova is the more scientifically correct medical term, we will use the colloquial terminology of egg/eggs, which is common to the medical profession, the press, and most lay people.

a quantum leap in social and psychological complexity. Couples choose this option with varying degrees of understanding of the possible future consequences.

• As couples experience repeated treatment failures, they begin to despair of ever having a genetically related child. The Resolution phase, comprised of three overlapping subphases, involves *ending medical treatment*, acknowledging and *mourning* the loss of not having a genetically related child, and *refocusing* on other possibilities in life, such as adoption or life without children.

• The Legacy phase encompasses the aftermath of the experience with infertility. Marital, sexual, and parenting problems may emerge as a consequence of the infertility, particularly when partners have not adequately handled the significant losses accompanying this experience. On the other hand, postinfertile parents often bring a maturity and commitment to parenting because of the difficulties they have encountered. Although sadness tends to be a lingering legacy, those couples who have been able to face this hardship together often find their marriages have been strengthened.

2

‏&‎

TREATMENT OVERVIEW

Although we give detailed suggestions for treatment in each phase in this book, this chapter covers the therapeutic principles that guide our work.

THE IMPORTANCE OF LANGUAGE

In our introduction, we discussed our preference for using the term "struggling with infertility" rather than the label "infertile." This semantic choice, based on White and Epston's (1990) concept of *externalizing the problem,* permits a shift in the couple's experiences from a passive posture of *being* infertile to a more active stance of *struggling* with infertility.

In sessions, we are likely to discuss this preference with each couple and explain why we prefer to talk about "struggling with infertility." We suggest that if they choose, they may want to adopt this language as their own. At first, the change often seems awkward. In time, however, couples and clinicians alike often find that this phrasing becomes increasingly effortless, and subtle changes can occur in how couples experience the condition and themselves.

Another benefit that results from externalizing the problem with infertility, a condition in which, typically, only one partner carries the infertility factor, is that the phrase "We are struggling with infertility" suggests that it is not so much the carrier but the infertility that provides the challenge for the couple. This semantic frame, which puts less onus on the carrier, may also unite and position the couple to act as a team in

16

their encounters with infertility. We have noticed that this language shift can lead to a cognitive change that, in turn, seems to defuse the tension and reduce the levels of guilt and blame insofar as carrier status is concerned.

Faye described it this way:

> "I used to get really depressed thinking, 'It just wasn't fair. I wasn't infertile, he was.' And I'd get really resentful and angry, and even feel guilty thinking this. I was getting really upset all the time thinking this. . . . I don't get so caught up in 'It's his fault' these days. The way I look at it is, we're both battling this thing."

A second issue connected to language that we have faced in working with this population is choosing a term to describe the couple's state of being without children. As we discussed in the introduction, the two commonly used choices, "childless" and "childfree," have very different implications, neither of which captures the attitude toward children held by most couples who struggle with infertility: "I have read all the books on infertility and I know the lingo—there are many days when I see myself as a childfree woman, but there are also days when I feel 'childless.' "

Our solution in practice has been to discuss the choice of labels with couples, and ask them which one—if any—fits the way they feel and think about themselves. While the term "involuntary childlessness" is gaining currency in the medical arena, couples have preferred such phrases as "We are a couple struggling to have a baby," "We are a couple without children," or simply, "We don't have kids yet." This often leads to an exploration of the ways in which infertility is seen by our culture. However, no matter what term a couple elects, our intention in addressing the issue of labels is to place couples in a position that allows them to experience greater distance from their infertility and to have the sense that it is a "for now" experience, not a fixed identity.

In conducting our sessions, we focus on the kinds of questions that help people to discover the various meanings they attribute to their experience with infertility. In this regard, the questions become interventions in and of themselves. *Meaning* encompasses the premises, assumptions, beliefs, paradigms, and myths that frame most, if not all, experience. These internal constructions are experienced as "reality"; they influence how people perceive internal and external events, how they determine which information is selected as relevant or ignored, and how people make assumptions about the intentions of others.

Because infertility evokes several interconnected assumptions about one's masculinity or femininity, parenthood, the value and meaning of children, and even the meaning of life, this kind of questioning can be most useful. Couples are likely to discover "problematic premises"—that is, premises that constrict options, limit possibilities, and constrain people to view themselves and their partners in a negative light. In such cases, we are likely to ask interventive questions (Tomm, 1987a, 1987b, 1987c).

These are questions that (1) invite couples to locate the familial and cultural expectations and mandates that influence their beliefs, and to think about how such beliefs may have originated; (2) encourage couples to consider new ways of perceiving their experiences; (3) allow them both to clarify their conflicts with each other and to locate their shared beliefs; (4) elicit their sense of power and control; and (5) provide couples with an opportunity to envision futures in which alternative scenarios are possible. In the course of asking interventive questions, the semantic separation between the infertility and the couple is maintained.

RESPECT AND LIMIT THE IMPACT OF INFERTILITY

Infertility Is Primary

Although this book focuses on therapy with couples, it is important for the clinician to remind him- or herself that a couple's encounter with infertility is not entirely negative. As a result of the challenge of infertility, couples may find ways of functioning more collaboratively, discovering hidden resources, improving their communication, resolving conflicts more effectively, and feeling more sympathetic toward each other. Many also take advantage of the opportunity to explore their interior selves in order to discover their life goals, core beliefs, philosophies, and world views related to children. More than one couple has called this odyssey the "silver lining" of their ordeal.

In the midst of their struggle with infertility, many others recognize that although they would like to rise to meet the challenge of infertility, they need help. But even in these circumstances, partners may not appreciate how much the infertility—rather than the other partner, themselves, or even their relationships—gives rise to their difficulties. The more couples are caught in the tangle of difficulties that accompany infertility and its treatments, the more they come to identity themselves as "infertile" and the less they see or appreciate other qualities and attributes. Therefore, we have found it helpful to encourage couples to stand back from their experiences with infertility and see the many ways in which this harrowing ordeal has come to define them, how the infertility has intruded upon their lives, altered their view of themselves and the world, and placed exceptional demands on their relationship.

The Phases of Infertility chapters that follow describe the progression of stressors and the effects on each partner and the relationship. As we work with couples we help them identify infertility's influence:

- Infertility may threaten one's identity, and often succeeds in making people feel physically defective, less feminine or masculine, less capable, and even ill-fated.
- Infertility puts the couple's future on hold by stalling their passage into the childrearing phase of their life. This limbo usually affects their emotional lives, and may affect—in more practical terms—their status in their families and the world at large.
- Medicine's remarkable new technologies—particularly in the area of donors and surrogates—may also produce biopsychosocial configurations never before imagined, whose outcomes cannot be predicted.
- Last, but definitely not least, infertility produces a significant drain on the couple's resources by exacting a great deal of time, money, and emotional energy. As a result, couples are deprived of the everyday pleasures and activities that support and replenish couple life.

In the process of spotlighting infertility's power, we remind couples that it is a formidable adversary and suggest that the best stance to take is one in which they remember to separate themselves—as individuals and as a couple—from the infertility.

Telling the Story

We introduce the importance of understanding infertility's influence early in the therapeutic engagement with the couple. No matter which phase they are in, once it becomes clear that they are dealing with infertility, we ask them to tell us about their struggle. Many couples in the Mobilization and Immersion phases begin by talking about the unique characteristics of their diagnoses including medical procedures that have been tried and the failures that resulted. For others, the narrative begins at the Dawning phase when the reality of what they were facing began to emerge. Or it might be the most recent couple conflict or treatment failure that begins the story, for example, a failed procedure or a miscarriage, or a couple's impasse about continuing medical interventions.

Stories about their medical experiences and relationships with infertility specialists are frequently at the core of couples' narratives. Because their medical expertise regarding reproduction and infertility medicine is very sophisticated, we urge therapists to acquaint themselves with the basic diagnoses, procedures, and medications (see the Appendix). Couples are gratified to be spared having to explain the complex alphabet soup of procedures. Furthermore, the clinician's familiarity with the various treatment protocols, medications, symptoms, and side effects provides the basis for understanding a significant component of the infertility ordeal. However, if the clinician is just beginning to acquire information about infertility and its treatments, he or she can ask the couple to explain the medical terminology or condition. This is certainly preferable to remaining in the dark or steering the session to more familiar (psychological) ground.

Many couples report that this therapy is the first time that they have told their story, together as a couple, and been encouraged to speak about the medical, emotional, and relational aspects of the experience. Often, one partner has become the historian or narrator, and because this limits the perspective on the encounter, we are careful to be sure that both partners are involved in telling the story. This may mean halting one partner's narrative to ask the other about his or her thoughts and feelings about the particular event.

LAURA: When the doctor gave us all the test results and he said that my getting pregnant was going to be hard, maybe out of the question entirely . . . I just felt like I was spinning, falling, dizzy, and I couldn't get my breath back. My heart was pounding, I couldn't think; it was like my mind just froze. It was like the worst day of my life. . . . It was a really long time before I could think of anything else.

CLINICIAN: Gene, what was that moment like for you? Did it hit you the same way?

GENE: Not really, my mind was somewhere else. I wasn't really taking the whole thing so seriously, like I wasn't really facing up to the fact that this was really a problem.

CLINICIAN: When did it register, you know, really sink in for you?

GENE: I guess by the time of the second one [failed medical procedure]. Then I knew we were really up against something here; she wasn't crazy.

Not only is the gathering of information about experiences with infertility vital to a clinician's understanding, but the telling itself is a necessary therapeutic step that helps couples step out of the current predicament and take a look at the various ways in which infertility has engulfed their lives. It is also a time for each partner to hear about what the other partner has been experiencing as the ordeal persisted.

In eliciting the story, the clinician might also ask the partners how the infertility has affected their relationships with their families, friends, and colleagues. Notice, in the next portion of the interview, how the clinician extends the narrative to include the way in which changes between the partners altered the wife's relationship with her mother.

CLINICIAN: *(to Laura)* Did you realize that it was taking Gene longer to see what you were up against?

LAURA: Not really, no. I just thought he didn't really care as much as I did.

CLINICIAN: And, what was it like before you and Laura were at the same place, you know, before you both could see how serious a problem the infertility was?

GENE: Well, like in the beginning, I couldn't help feeling she was getting hysterical over nothing—or maybe not really nothing, but something that wasn't such a big deal.

CLINICIAN: And so, tell me, what were things like between you two then, you know, back before you were both looking at the infertility in the same way?

LAURA: At the time, you mean? Well, I guess if I look back now I gotta say we weren't very close.

GENE: Like *really* not close. She was always mad at me, and I was trying to stay away from her altogether.

LAURA: I'd be crying all night, and he'd just turn over in bed, or go into the living room and watch TV all night.

CLINICIAN: Did you find someone else to talk to during that time?

LAURA: My mother and I talked a lot. . . . We got very close, she was right there for me. She still is.

The Community of Others: Normalizing the Infertility

Because couples have often withdrawn from their social networks hoping to avoid the painful feelings of deviance and shame generated by child-focused gatherings, they often feel isolated. Although we try to help couples understand the role that cultural attitudes have in generating these feelings, such awareness may do little to remedy the sense of being an outsider.

When our project first began, we realized that couples coping with infertility were feeling isolated and alienated, as evidenced by the nearly universal appreciation couples expressed toward our team for creating the Infertility Project.[1] "It means we're not alone, doesn't it?" said one woman.

Although not all clinicians are in the fortunate position of being able to work with a team that specializes in couples struggling with infertility, clinicians can talk about the experiences of others with couples in the course of their treatment and, in this way, create a community of others who also struggle with infertility. A standard part of our protocol is to ask couples if we might have their permission to share with others facing infertility any useful coping strategies they have devised (with the proviso, of course, that their identities are kept confidential). As a way of introducing the notion of the community of other couples, we might say something along the following lines:

> "I thought you might want to know about some ways others have coped with [the particular challenge the couple is facing]. These are not the only ways or the best ways, but just the kinds of solutions others have found helpful. They might work for you, or give you a running start in being able to think about how you might handle this situation. After all, many couples in your position are making things up as they go along. In a sense you are forced into being pioneers and might benefit from those who are a little ahead of you on the road. And, if you find a useful way of dealing with a problem, and you feel comfortable with letting me pass it on to others like yourselves, I am sure they would appreciate it."

This approach contrasts sharply with traditional psychotherapy, and it often surprises couples who come expecting that the clinician will be circumspect and adhere to traditional psychotherapeutic practices. When the clinician refers to a kindred community, in addition to couples' feeling less isolated, they are provided with a channel for sharing their successes and are thereby given the opportunity to turn their struggle into a valuable resource for others.

In one instance, a couple considered another couple's strategy for coping with family gatherings, but did not find the approach appropriate for their particular situation. However, they took comfort in knowing that there were others who were trying to cope with similar difficulties. In discussing why another couple's solutions did not fit them, they discovered a better solution for themselves. Introducing couples to RESOLVE, a national self-help and information group, is another way of providing community (see Chapter 8).

---

[1]Pauline Boss, who has done ground-breaking research on ambiguous loss (1991), visited our project and suggested that by serving as witnesses to the experience of infertility, the team was providing couples with a sense of community.

Scheduling Appointments

The stresses and challenges of infertility vary from couple to couple and from time to time with each couple. Sometimes a couple is in crisis, whereas at other times things are more stable. Therefore, we suggest that clinicians work with couples to fine-tune the scheduling of their sessions. At the beginning of treatment, we state that we do not assume that scheduling appointments weekly, bimonthly, or at any fixed interval will always fit the changing demands of infertility. Many couples come with expectations based on standard psychotherapeutic protocols and assume that sessions will occur weekly; therefore, we point out that the course of each couple's experience with infertility is different and often erratic, and suggest that they may wish to schedule sessions to fit with their own needs. We believe that couples often know best whether longer or shorter spacing is appropriate; no two couples have elected the same kinds of scheduling, although most prefer weekly or biweekly meetings during the beginning of treatment.

An added benefit of placing the scheduling of appointments in the couple's hands is that we are giving couples a greater sense of control over their lives. This becomes another way of reinforcing the idea that problems arise from coping with infertility, not from the couple's relationship per se. For example, when one couple was perplexed about whether to proceed with a donor insemination, three sessions were held within a 10-day period. Another couple, pregnant and "just waiting for time to go by and not wanting to tempt the gods" by discussing their anxious anticipation, preferred a 4-week break before meeting again.

Empowerment

Giving couples power in terms of scheduling appointments is one of several ways the clinician may want to address the profound out-of-control feelings that permeate the infertility. Abbey, Halman, and Andrews (1992) found that the more out of control people feel, the greater their distress, and conversely, the more people feel they have control, the less their distress. Although part of coping with infertility is acknowledging its power and one's feeling of powerlessness, it is just as important to remind people that they are not entirely helpless.

THE THERAPEUTIC TRIANGLE

In working with couples struggling with infertility, we have found it useful to think about three separate but interrelated areas: the couples, their infertility, and ourselves, the clinicians. We call this the *therapeutic triangle*.

Infertility is seen as a precipitating crisis that if prolonged, develops into a chronic condition. Like many acute and chronic crises, infertility seems to find both the stronger and weaker points in the couple's relationship and to bring them into the foreground. In this regard, we metaphorically liken infertility to a plow that unearths all manner of coping strategies, belief systems, and personal and couple histories: "I would say that any problems that were there—even sort of nascent problems that maybe never would have come into full bloom—have all been brought to the surface because of this."

For the clinician and the couple, teasing apart problems within the partners' relationship and those related to their struggle with infertility becomes the central focus of treatment. Sometimes it is helpful to look at what is going on with the couple through the lens of infertility, and sometimes it is helpful to look at how the couple is handling the infertility through the lens of the couple's relationship. By alternating these lenses, a clearer picture emerges of both the couple and the infertility.

The clinician must also bear in mind that he or she has a lens, a perspective, a host of beliefs and attitudes that are likely to influence the picture of the couple that emerges. If we are to help couples look at, understand, and cope with their infertility, we must pay attention to what we ourselves think and feel about children, parenthood, and infertility. Just as we suggest that couples explore why and how they came to their feelings and beliefs, so we must examine our own. Along these lines, we look at our family beliefs, the choices we have made about children and parenting, why and how we made them, and how these may relate to our thoughts about our clients. Paying attention to this third side of the therapeutic triangle—ourselves—can be the most difficult in that conscientious self-examination requires a steady vigilance.

One way we try to track our preferences and attitudes is to ask ourselves questions such as "Why am I leaning more toward the partner who wants to try another procedure?" "Why do I feel that one partner is being unfair in insisting on another child?" "Why do I think they are giving up too soon/persevering too long?" "Am I mistaking motherhood for womanhood? Fertility for masculinity?" The longer we work with couples, the more we find that although our assumptions, beliefs, and biases have not necessarily changed, they are more accessible to our conscious scrutiny. As a result, we tend to be more careful about inadvertently influencing people to embrace our beliefs and the choices that are the logical outcomes of those beliefs. However, when significant differences appear between our beliefs and those of our clients, and we think that these differences may have an impact on the therapy, we are likely to discuss our perspective and its origins with the couples.

> One of us worked with an Orthodox Jewish couple who had four children, and were part of a Hasidic community in which it was usual for parents to have much larger families. Naomi and Jeremy had planned to have "six, seven, maybe more children." Naomi had undergone several infertility protocols involving surgeries and numerous cycles of hormone injections. The couple had nearly exhausted their savings and were thinking about taking out loans for the next procedure. Naomi had been in the care of an infertility specialist for 5 years when she called the therapist because she had become so depressed that she could not function and was neglecting her children. Jeremy was working overtime to support the family and pay the medical bills, and was not able to assist in childcare.
>
> After meeting with the couple for several weeks, the clinician began to question the couple's insistence on continuing infertility protocols while their children were being neglected. She raised these worries with Naomi and Jeremy saying that she too was Jewish, and like them, came from a family that placed a high value on children and parenting. However, in her family, the quality of parenting seemed to be more important than the number of children. Therefore, she told them, she was having a hard time understanding why they were insisting on more children if it meant that those children they did have might be neglected.
>
> What followed, by way of explanation, was a moving account of how each of their families had lost many relatives in the Holocaust. Furthermore, their particular sect placed great importance on having large families. Therefore, following this particular mandate was a way of preserving the values that they and their deceased relatives had embraced.
>
> The clinician was then able to join with the couple and talk about how parents raise children to observe their religion, honor their ancestors, and conserve the spiritual legacy of each of their families. Naomi and Jeremy began to concentrate more on the four children they did have. With this refocusing, the infertility treatments were moved to a back burner, and after several months the couple discontinued medical interventions.

THE PHASES OF INFERTILITY: LOCATE THE COUPLE ON THE TRAJECTORY

Because there is generally a progression of phases through which couples pass during their struggle with infertility, we find it useful to locate couples on the trajectory through the stages. This phase-specific perspective is helpful in understanding a couple's struggles and planning clinical interventions. Additionally, there are times when couples can benefit from information about a specific phase. However, in our clinical work, we do not offer couples a discourse on the phases of infertility, nor do we assume that each couple's passage will be the same. Instead, when we notice that couples are encountering obstacles, feelings, or decisions that others have faced, we may talk about the experiences of others in terms of phase specificity. This serves both as way of orienting couples to aspects of the phase they are in and providing couples with the sense of community mentioned above, in that it provides a fellowship with other couples who have traveled a similar route.

Although older couples, whose fertility rates decline more rapidly than younger couples, are likely to view time as their enemy, even younger couples dread the future when viewed through the lens of infertility. A life without children looms as a frightening specter. However, when couples avoid thinking of the future, a sense of limbo can stymie their ability to make decisions and take actions that will hold up over time. Any discussion we have with couples about the phases and trajectory of infertility serves as a reminder of the future—something that couples are likely to lose sight of during the limbo of infertility and its treatments. In talking with the couple about what might happen next in terms of phases, we gradually extend the conversation to include what lies on the horizon. We find that couples eventually gain comfort in confronting their fears or what lies ahead. And furthermore, if we fast forward to the future (Penn, 1985) and discuss what couples would like to see for themselves, what legacies they would want to leave, we can effectively introduce a discussion of children and parenting, covered later in this chapter.

THE FOCUS ON THE COUPLE RELATIONSHIP

Coping with infertility and its treatments can be so overwhelming that couples are likely to neglect their personal lives and their relationship. At first, couples make these sacrifices in response to the immediate crisis infertility presents. As months or years of failed attempts to get pregnant pass, there is less time, energy, and incentive to have fun and enjoy each other's company. Yet, not unexpectedly, to cope with day-to-day stresses, couples need to invest a share of their time and energy in preserving their relationship.

In order to address this dilemma—that is, nourishing the relationship in the face of infertility—we help couples protect or, if necessary, rediscover ways of spending time together as a couple separate from the infertility and its treatments. We suggest cordoning off or creating areas in their lives that can serve as infertility-free, safe havens. When it comes to the practical management of infertility itself, we encourage couples to function as a team. These two aspects—infertility-free time together and teamwork when handling the infertility—are interrelated: The more robust the relationship, the better the teamwork; the better the teamwork, the greater the motivation to enjoy time together.

The First Meeting

By the time partners decide that they need therapy, their relationship may be showing severe signs of wear. Because struggling with infertility "always feels like a losing battle" and the emotional toll is extreme, the couple is rarely able to address the many problems that arise, and there may be a backlog of problems and concerns. Partners are likely to display the kinds of symptoms typically present when seeking couple therapy. However, the degree of conflict or disaffection may be so great that the clinician often has serious concerns about how helpful couple therapy can be. Furthermore, he or she may mistakenly read the signs of protracted distress over infertility as pathological and refer one or both partners for individual therapy. This is less likely to happen with clinicians who are familiar with this cohort of couples. Although there are certainly situations in which either of these clinical assessments may be correct, in our work we tend to find that for many couples, after relatively few sessions, there is a marked decrease in both individual distress and couple tension.

A clinician's misreading of the distress as overreaction is most likely to occur during the Immersion phase when the acute distress is most evident. However, it is also possible that an inexperienced clinician might assume that the degree of distress shown by couples in the early phases is somehow out of proportion to the stressor, whereas during the later phases, the stressors are more obvious. Unless infertility is mentioned in the history, its role in the picture of the couple that emerges may be obscured altogether. One clinician, new to the field and inexperienced at understanding and dealing with infertility, said, "After all, it's just infertility, it's not a life-threatening illness!"

Individual or Couple Therapy?

After couples have spent considerable time and energy dealing with the infertility, individual partners are likely to make the obvious connection between their personal distress and the infertility. However, they may assume that the best way to alleviate their distress is through individual therapy. Because women are the primary, if not sole, patients in the medical arena, they may see psychotherapy as an essential adjunct to coping with infertility and its treatments. Furthermore, because women may be more likely than men to want to talk about their difficulties and may even have tried speaking with their partners with little success, they may stake out the therapeutic territory for themselves. Men often feel that they are helpless and peripheral insofar as the infertility is concerned, and they may therefore feel relieved when their partners seek help from a professional.

Individually oriented therapists may agree that individual therapy is the most productive way to proceed with problems around infertility. In support of this position, they cite an individual's reluctance to speak freely in couple sessions for fear of hurting their partners or damaging the relationship. They believe that without feeling comfortable to explore the range of feelings that are part of the infertility experience, the therapeutic work will be compromised.

Systemic therapists believe that the clinician who accepts the individual therapy request may inadvertently be creating an added problem for the couple. Whether the client is a man or a woman, the clinician is likely to become a surrogate partner in coping with the infertility. Without making the missing partner a member of the team, problems between the partners are not only likely to persist but may worsen. As with any problem that crops up in a couple's life, when one partner is left out of the solution, and a third person is recruited into solving the problem, rifts in the couple's relationship can widen.

We have found that when one partner contacts the clinician for therapy, when the clinician raises the idea of meeting with both partners, there is usually a willingness to do so, at least for one session. At these initial meetings, it is not uncommon for men to state that because their distress is less than their partners, they feel helpless and hope that their partner will eventually become the primary patient. Similarly, a woman may bring her mate to the first session in order to show the clinician what she is up against insofar as her partner's limitations when it comes to understanding her distress. But once the process begins, both partners are usually able to understand the interactive aspect of coping with infertility, and both are likely to see the relevance of continuing in couple therapy.

Another way in which a couple may present for therapy is when the partners are in conflict about an important decision such as whether to repeat or end medical interventions, elect or reject donor gametes, begin the adoption process, or proceed without children. They hope to use the therapist as a mediator in order to help them to resolve the present impasse. For such couples, because the difficulty in reaching a mutually agreeable decision may be symptomatic of other problems that have been accumulating during the ordeal with infertility, it is important that the therapist help the couple review the events that have led them to this decision by asking the couple to tell the story of their infertility. Although they may at first be impatient with or resistant to this idea, once the initial meeting is underway, the couple may feel less concerned about arriving at an immediate solution to their impasse and more concerned with the larger picture, their relationship.

Teamwork and the Management of the Infertility

We encourage partners to attend medical appointments together whenever feasible. In particular, when one partner is alone—either at home or at work—and receives news that a procedure has failed, his or her sense of isolation is intensified. We therefore stress the importance of trying to be together whenever they are expecting to receive significant medical information such as phone calls from physicians regarding pregnancy and embryo transfer results. Even conference calls to physicians are preferable to one partner having to face the news alone. Being with each other at crucial information-receiving occasions is an essential part of the practical and emotional partnership necessary to cope with infertility and its treatments. Couples can share the joy of good news, or give and receive comfort when the news is bad.

The clinician can initially, and then periodically, encourage these kinds of cooperative efforts and work with the couple to lighten the emotional load of the partner who has been carrying most of the treatment burden. The clinician can help couples find ways of joining together against the infertility instead of pulling apart or against each other.

Highlighting the importance of functioning as a team is helpful to couples during Dawning and Mobilization when couples are just beginning to deal with infertility. During these phases, they may perceive infertility as though it were no different than any other medical condition in that both partners do not, as a rule, visit doctors together. However, by the time couples are in Immersion, most have either understood the benefits of teamwork or are feeling the drawbacks of working unilaterally. After discussing the disadvantages of any problematic patterns, new strategies can be discussed and planned.

For situations in which couples enter therapy during the later stages of their ordeal with infertility, there is, of course, far less need to highlight the cooperative handling of medical issues, and more need to focus on mourning losses together and planning for the future. Recovering from the ordeal of infertility is enhanced by a climate of mutual understanding and compassion; therefore, it is also helpful to encourage couples to recollect all the crises they weathered together, to take stock of their strengths, recognize the weaker areas of functioning that were revealed during the stresses of infertility, and think about how to improve these coping areas in the future.

Teamwork in the Clinician's Office

In sessions, the clinician helps the couple to focus on both partners' experiences. For example, if the woman describes the ordeal she experienced during a medical procedure, the clinician can ask her partner what he was thinking and feeling during that time. Although the actual experiences are usually very different, and men are rarely the patients receiving the various medical interventions, their feelings and thoughts about infertility and the particular medical intervention can be just as intense as those of their partners. However, men often feel that it is unfair to share their worries and distress with their partners because the women are already bearing most of the physical inconvenience (or outright suffering) associated with testing and treatments.

At the start of treatment, for the reasons stated above, men may feel awkward when asked to talk about their experiences. However, once they begin they are likely to appreciate the opportunity. Women may be surprised and gratified to learn that their partners have been so concerned about and invested in dealing with the infertility: "It helps me to know he's there, even if it's just him worrying on the sidelines," said one woman. With another couple, after a husband sobbed openly about the couple's numerous failures to conceive, he was surprised at his wife's empathic response. He said, "I've been so scared to break down in front of you [his wife]. I kept thinking the thing to do was to be strong." His wife said, "When I'm the one that's always breaking down, I never get the chance to be the strong one, to comfort you. . . . I can't seem to do such a really simple thing—just have a baby—something everybody else can do. At least let me be a wife. Let me be there for you."

On the other hand, when men have been forthcoming about their distress, particularly when they are carriers of the infertility factor, women may censor any of their own expression of distress. One husband, for example, a carrier of the infertility factor, had little difficulty articulating his pain and suffering. His wife felt she had no right to speak with him about her pain because she was not the carrier, and she tried to restrain any show of emotion. With a second couple, a more typical pattern emerged: the wife was the carrier and her husband felt that to show his grief and disappointment would have felt like a rebuke to his wife. Although the clinician's efforts to externalize the infertility can dispel some of the onus associated with carrier status, an open airing of each partner's feelings about the issue is equally important.

In general, our method is one that helps couples approach the painful issues that infertility raises, issues that have been avoided for fear of injuring the other, the self, or the relationship. This is especially important for couples who appear to be functioning as a team, but whose cohesion is based on an implicit rallying cry of "us against them." Although they may derive great unity from this kind of alliance, their tacit contract is to avoid injuring each other above all else. Talking about painful thoughts and feelings, especially those associated with carrier and noncarrier status, is seen as a threat to the couple's cohesion. Difficult areas are typically unspoken, denied, or glossed over.

The "us against them" strategy seems to work well in the short run, but we have noticed that it becomes decreasingly effective as time goes by. First, it can take over other areas of their lives, polarizing relationships with friends and family. Second, each partner may find it increasingly difficult to suppress thoughts and feelings that might cause the other pain or discomfort. Either the fragile wall of silence may crumble and the pent-up disappointments and resentments related to the infertility pour forth, or one or both may withdraw from the other. In either case, secrecy creates a less than propitious emotional environment in which to introduce a child.

Separate Sessions: Speaking the Unspeakable

When we first began to see couples in separate sessions as part of our project's treatment protocol, we found it so fruitful that we now hold separate sessions more often in our work with other couples, not just those struggling with infertility. We find that the "unspeakable" themes evoked by the infertility are likely to result in uncertainty and guardedness about what to share with one's partner. Couples need a forum in which to express these thoughts, feelings, and fantasies, to "speak the unspeakable."

Early in our meetings with couples, we state that our way of working is couple focused, but that this does not always mean that both partners must be present at all sessions. We tell couples that we usually schedule a separate meeting with each partner within the first few weeks of therapy. We also encourage couples to let us know whenever they think this kind of meeting might be useful to them. Sometimes we can sense that one or both partners are having great difficulty speaking in sessions, and so we ask whether it feels like a good time for a set of individual sessions. To date, each time we have raised the possibility, couples have concurred.

We inform couples that these meetings provide a protected arena to talk about difficult matters that seem uncomfortable to express in the couple sessions. We explain that our goal is to help partners bring back to the couple meetings important issues that were discussed during the separate sessions and bear on the couple's relationship.

At the separate sessions, partners typically require little urging to talk about the feelings and thoughts that trouble them the most. However, although most partners find it easy to focus in on those areas, others may have difficulty articulating their distress and their overwhelming feelings of sadness, anger, jealousy, fear, shame, and blame. Often their silence about these feelings is geared toward trying to protect themselves and their partners from pain and conflict, rather than toward keeping secrets from their partners.

Feelings not only about the partner, but about the self are likely to be discussed. Carriers may not feel comfortable discussing feelings of shame, defect, or decreased sense of sexual desirability with their partners. Noncarriers may suppress negative thoughts and feelings related to their mates. Normalizing some of the reactions people have toward themselves or their partners is useful to a degree, especially because we are all subject to the effects of the cultural attitudes that link fertility with femininity, masculinity, motherhood, and fatherhood. However, it is equally important for the clinician to explore and challenge these beliefs in the ways described later in this chapter.

Although not necessarily typical, fantasies of leaving, ending the relationship, and having a baby with another partner can arise. These fantasies may cause the clinician to worry that she or he is opening a Pandora's box by holding separate meetings, but we find that talking with a professional about these thoughts and feelings, normalizing them, and exploring the assumptions that lie beneath these notions appears to render them less damaging and can diminish their intensity. The clinician and partner can then talk about what material might be useful to take back to the conjoint session, and what might be left unsaid. Partners may choose to talk with their mates about the issues, or the material may be neutralized to the point where it no longer holds the power it had had before being discussed with the clinician. When partners elect to keep significant feelings and thoughts secret, and not discuss them with their partners, the consequences of talking or not talking with the partner are explored.

> Phyllis told us in a separate session that she did not want to have sex with her husband, Glenn, because he was sterile. She no longer found him sexy, and sex was a painful reminder of what they could not do, that is, make a baby. She preferred faking it sexually rather

than tell him because she feared it would hurt him and hurt their relationship. She felt these things were best shared with her individual therapist.

We asked her whether, if the situation were reversed, she would want him to tell her. She said, "Absolutely not!" We then asked her, "How do you imagine your marriage will be in the future if you take all your painful issues to an individual therapist rather than to your husband?"

At the next couple session, Phyllis spoke about how she had thought about what we said and decided to speak with Glenn. She was amazed to discover that he, too, was finding sex a painful and unpleasant reminder.

In working with individuals around infertility it is important to notice the extent to which clients' feelings about themselves, their partners, and the relationship remain in the therapy, and what is shared with the partner.

If a partner leans toward, but is apprehensive about, bringing material to the couple session, the clinician can work with the individual to find a compassionate way of talking to the absent partner about what was raised in session. Loss of sexual passion, for example, is a common problem that partners tend not to discuss with each other. Learning from the clinician that this is a common complaint for couples who have spent a long time trying to get pregnant may make it a less difficult topic to discuss with one's partner. Because it is quite likely that the partner who is not at the session feels the same way about the sex, we suggest that each partner start by acknowledging his or her sadness about having to sacrifice spontaneous sexual pleasure. The aim is not only to try to prevent further erosion of their sexual life, but to prevent it from spilling over into other areas of couple intimacy. Fixing or reversing the problem (see Chapter 14) takes more effort, and the couple may not be ready to approach it until after they have produced a child, adopted, or chosen to live without children.

Taking Time Out from Infertility

The landscape of infertility is filled with disappointment, failure, and feelings of blame, shame, and personal defect. Therefore, the challenge for the clinician is to help couples reestablish areas of their lives that give them pleasure and provide respite from infertility and its treatments. This can be difficult because, suspended in the limbo of infertility, couples are likely to have moved away from other relationships or dropped out of many of the activities that had been part of their former lives. Infertility not only becomes a preoccupation but confines the couple to an increasingly constricted environment. "It feels as though our life has shrunk," said one man. "It's infertility and nothing else."

One of the clinician's roles can be that of lobbyist, exploring what has interfered with the couple's ability to engage in non-infertility-related activities. Then, he or she might strongly encourage the couple to put more of these activities back into their lives. The clinician can raise the possibility of having infertility-free days or suspending treatments from time to time. On infertility-free days, suggested "homework" might be having dinner out, going away for a weekend, meeting for lunch, and other mutually enjoyable activities.

> It was serendipitous that Frank and Cheryl ran into traffic problems on the way to our clinic, and, by the time they arrived, they had only 20 minutes remaining in their scheduled session. Unable to meet because another couple was scheduled for the next hour, the clinician suggested that the couple take the fee they were to have spent on the session and go to lunch at a special restaurant. At the following session, the couple talked about how pleasantly surprised they had been to find they could still enjoy themselves. "We remembered how much fun we used to have in places like this. . . . It was romantic . . . not something we would have thought to do on our own, not since this [the infertility] all began," said Cheryl. "So, we decided we just have to do more stuff like this." However, although they agreed that putting fun back in their lives was vital, the clinician periodically had to ask how that part of their life was going, and humorously chide them when they forgot to do their homework.

Sex for Baby Making versus Sex for Fun

Although problems in the areas of arousal and performance can occur with any couple, these sexual difficulties are common to couples who face infertility. Most come to accept the fact that spontaneous sex, engaged in simply for pleasure, cannot be sustained when concerns about pregnancy dominate.

The clinician who has not worked with couples struggling with infertility may regard the loss of sexual pleasure, which sometimes even becomes an aversion toward sex, as symptomatic of more profound couple problems. One clinician, for example, who consulted the team about a couple who spoke nonchalantly about their "mechanical sex," assumed that the partners "lacked intimacy." However, for couples whose sex life has been impacted by the ordeal of infertility, the reverse may be true: As one couple put it, "Being intimate *without* having good sex is proof of *real* intimacy."

Sometimes couples will present for treatment when one partner is far more unhappy with the absence of a pleasurable sex life than his or her mate. In these instances, tension develops between partners about the relative importance of good sex versus getting pregnant. When sex and baby making are pitted against each other, the partners can become embroiled in polarized struggles. For these couples, we find it useful to take a "both-and" position. We honor the logic of both partners' positions: While one keeps an eye on family making, the other keeps an eye on making sure the couple's relationship, which will become a child's primary universe, will endure and flourish. We raise the idea of taking periodic breaks from baby-making sex, and reinstating sex for fun. For some this may only entail initiating sex at times when there is no chance of fertilization occurring. For others, it means taking days or weeks off from infertility protocols; we call this *sabbaticals from treatment.*

The notion of suspension of treatment, however, is difficult for many who want the ordeal of infertility to end. It is especially problematic for older couples who fear that time is running out and they must use every opportunity to try to get pregnant. Infertility specialists, whose focus is on helping couples have babies, are likely to reinforce these couples' sense of urgency and not "wasting" time. It is, indeed, a difficult dilemma. The clinician can help the couple sort out the possible consequences of sacrificing enjoyable, spontaneous sex in order to get pregnant by asking them to consider the long- and short-term effects, the pluses and minuses of losing time versus preserving a place for love making.

EXPLORING COUPLES' BELIEF SYSTEMS

Infertility, the "plow" that thrusts itself through the couple's psychological field, unearths many cognitive constructions, world views, assumptions, premises, narratives, attributions, and explanations that are related to various aspects of infertility. These can collectively be called the couple's "beliefs."

The beliefs that dominate the territory of infertility are derived from a variety of sources. There are fairly universal notions that are part of the fabric of our society, as well as more specific ones that are common to one's ethnic or religious affiliation, class, gender, and multigenerational family and individual history. Lastly, there are also sets of shared beliefs generated by each couple during the years they spend together.

The couples' beliefs that become a part of the experience of infertility are not necessarily conscious or easily articulated, yet they are often assumed to be "truths," simply the way things are. They may include very basic notions such as "Children and marriage go together," "Fertility and masculinity are the same," "Women who cannot bear children are not *real* women," "Men who carry the infertility factor are not *real* men," or "Adopted children are always a problem." Idiosyncratic beliefs might include such constructs as infertility proves "I'm different," "I'm undeserving," "I'm less manly/womanly than others," or that "Nothing ever come easy for me and my family," or "Infertility is a sign that our union is flawed."

Some couples' beliefs help them get through the rougher waters of infertility. Examples of these are "Crises bring us together," or "If it doesn't kill you, it will make you stronger," or "The [family name]s can overcome all obstacles." More often, however, infertility elicits a host of beliefs that churn the emotional waters, making passage through the experience of infertility that much more difficult. We call the latter *problematic beliefs*.

Other couples hold beliefs that are not necessarily problematic in and of themselves, but become troublesome because there are conflicts in their convictions. Until a consensus is reached, whether by altering one or both partner's assumptions, finding a third frame that suits both, their ability to make sound decisions can be compromised.

Our approach in regard to problematic and conflicting beliefs is no different than with any population with whom we work. The first step is helping couples articulate their positions. Secondly, we work with each partner to find when, where, and how each view was learned and assimilated. The focus can then shift toward the exploration of alternatives, that is, other ways of understanding one's experience. Within this expanded discussion, the couple's universe of assumptions can widen and thereby yield a wider range of feelings, choices, and actions. We have found that there are basically four subdivisions of beliefs that tend to dominate the landscape of infertility: the *infertility* itself, assumptions about *maleness and femaleness*, the meaning and value of *children and parenting*, and the still unfamiliar territory of *donors*.

Infertility

First and foremost, fertility and infertility are likely to summon up associations about the masculinity and femininity of oneself and one's partner. Like other traumatic stressors in life, infertility taps into existential beliefs and world views. We repeatedly find that fertility is viewed as confirmation of worth, the reward for a virtuous life, and the marker of normality, whereas infertility is linked with an opposite set of ascriptions: less manliness or womanliness, confirmation of abnormality or worthlessness, and/or punishment for past wrongs. Themes of retribution for past misconduct, evidence of intrinsic inferiority, lack of entitlement, cause for shame, and the curse of perpetual bad luck are often linked with infertility: "These kinds of things always happen to me," "Why me? I don't deserve this." Conversely, "Why not me? I always fail, nothing in life ever comes easily for me," "Life sucks," "The world is unsafe," "I can't do anything right," and so forth.

In order to locate these beliefs, we start by asking the couple open-ended questions about the infertility such as "What does the diagnosis of infertility mean to you?" Some couples can immediately list a number of assumptions that have plagued them since the infertility was first diagnosed. Other couples, however, may feel embarrassed or ashamed of their seemingly absurd notions and may worry that the clinician will think their beliefs are "outdated" "stereotypical," or "irrational." Acknowledging this fear while asking more focused questions can be a more successful approach. For example, the clinician may want to preface the exploration of beliefs by saying, "Infertility is likely to stir up what may seem like totally fantastic, irrational thoughts and ideas. It's not uncommon for people facing infertility to have these thoughts. Do these kinds of ideas occur to each of you?"

Once couples feel comfortable talking about their beliefs, the clinician can then ask questions about the etiology of these constructs, that is, questions about how, when, and why they think these beliefs were generated. "Where do you think you learned that?" is a useful question. As it conveys the message that these ideas are not immutable, a priori "facts," it invites the listener to think about the means by which such ideas were imparted. These questions about derivation allow people to step back from their experience of infertility and appreciate the cultural, familial, and personal sources of their beliefs. In so doing, couples may have sufficient distance to question the immutability of their assumptions, to critique them, and to entertain the possibility of changing them. Questions might include some of the following:

- Where do you think you learned this?
- What are your ideas about how you came to think this?
- Have thoughts like these surfaced at other stressful times in your life? Or is there something special about infertility that evokes them?
- What kinds of messages does society give us about fertility and infertility?
- What ideas about infertility have you learned in your family? Are there any stories about family members who have experienced infertility?
- Is there some personal meaning that you attach to infertility?

- How do you think being a man/woman affects the way you are looking at this?

Such exploration can uncover problematic themes connected to the past. When asked about what past or current experiences might be affecting the way in which they view the infertility and the choices they have made, some individuals can immediately locate the sources.

> In answer to the question, "What has been most distressing to you about the infertility?" Teri, who had been born with a physical defect that had been corrected with surgery, said that she had never been able to reassure her parents or convince herself that she was as physically "normal" or "sturdy" as her siblings. Therefore, she felt that if she could conceive and give birth to a child, she would finally prove that her body was normal. For that reason she felt that adoption, her husband's first choice, was out of the question. She preferred donor insemination, a procedure that would give her the opportunity to demonstrate her physical normality.

For others, the blow to one's manhood or womanhood, or themes of physical defect are less pronounced. Instead, the most distressing part of the infertility is the loss of control. The themes of control and lack of control can then be probed.

> When asked why feeling out of control was so disturbing, Brad answered that he had always believed that he could maintain total control of his life: His father seemed to manage this feat effortlessly, and the capacity to be "in control at all times" was highly prized in his family. After much discussion, Brad was asked whether it would make sense to discuss this with his father. By doing so, Brad learned that his father's parents were totally out of control. Both paternal grandparents were alcoholics who were constantly fighting, losing jobs, and being evicted from their apartments. Realizing that the anxiety generated by loss of control was "not my story at all," Brad also realized that the infertility provided him with an arena in which to gain greater acceptance for that unavoidable human eventuality, feeling out of control.

Maleness and Femaleness

Because there is a considerable body of research concerning the differences in how men and women respond to and cope with the diagnosis and ordeal of infertility, we assume that although there may be hardwired differences between men and women, which may be difficult to alter, there are also gender-linked ideas that become a part of men's and women's socialization and may be more malleable. In order to avoid getting caught up in a debate about what is nature and what is nurture, we take the position that each perspective offers a way of understanding the differences that arise between men and women.

Researchers have studied the differences and similarities in the ways that men and women experience infertility. The following summary is presented with the caveat that the differences noted may reflect either nature or nurture, and that it is still important to discover why men and women in general, or any one particular couple, do or do not correspond to the overall average.

No matter which partner carries the infertility factor, women show greater pain than men: 50% of women and only 15% of men report that infertility is the most distressing experience of their lives (Freeman et al., 1985). As might be expected, compared to their partners, women have higher depression and anxiety scores. In addition, infertility has a more negative effect on women's satisfaction with life and sex, and their overall sense of well-being. (Andrews et al., 1992; Daniluk, 1988; Lalos, Lalos, Jacobsson, & Von Schultz, 1985; McEwan, Costello, & Taylor, 1987; Wright et al., 1991). Whereas both fertile women and those struggling with infertility experience high levels of distress, only men carrying the infertility factor report suffering that approximates that of women (Nachtigall, Becker, & Wozny, 1992).

Over time, men and women react differently to the diagnosis of infertility: Initially men are more optimistic, whereas women are far more disappointed, depressed, and despairing. Men tend to deny and distance themselves from the infertility; however, despite their withdrawal, they are likely to be more aware of their partner's reactions than they are of their own (Abbey et al., 1992; Greil, 1991; Mathews & Mathews, 1993; Wirtberg, 1992). Men who face infertility feel they have suffered a "blow to their virility," whereas women who face infertility describe themselves as "feeling incomplete" (Kraft et al., 1980).

Researchers who study gender distress (Abbey et al., 1992; Berg, Wilson, & Weingartner, 1991; Hendricks, 1985; Ulbrich, Tremaglio-Coyle, & Llabre, 1990), hypothesize that women's distress scores are higher because their identities and sense of self-worth are more likely to be linked not only to parenting, but also to producing a child. Men's distress, in comparison to women, increases as medical costs multiply. Abbey et al. (1992) ascribe this to men's concerns about the challenge infertility poses to their roles as providers.

Although men may appear to experience less distress, recent findings suggest that although men are less inclined to verbalize their feelings, their actual distress may be closer to their partners' (Berg et al., 1991). When the content, rather than the extent of the distress is ana-

lyzed, men and women appear to have similar responses to the infertility in the areas of role failure, loss and reduced self esteem (Nachtigall
et al., 1992); helplessness, guilt, inadequacy, and a focus on having a
child and a willingness to go to great lengths to do so, and descriptions of infertility as "the hardest part of my life" (Collins, Freeman,
Boxer, & Tureck, 1992). Over time, as men and women continue to
struggle with infertility, differences between them tend to decrease
(Berg & Wilson, 1991).

In general, our clinical experiences have supported this research.
Discussing gender-linked differences with couples can help partners to
understand each other, and to minimize conflicts that arise when one
partner tries to impose his or her feelings and attitudes on the other.

However, we are careful not to make any exploration of gender differences an occasion to endorse rigid gender stereotyping such that differences seem immutable and necessarily conflictual. Stereotyping, a
common part of the popular discourse, is likely to reinforce or even create barriers to couple intimacy. In addition to exploring each partner's
gender-related beliefs, we track how their beliefs were instilled and
shaped over time. Finally, we invite each to reexamine those beliefs to
see whether they can be changed.

In the course of our work with this population, although we tend to
find couples whose gender-related beliefs are consistent with researchers'
findings, there have also been notable exceptions, that is, men and
women who do not fit the gender stereotypes insofar as how they see
themselves in relation to the infertility and parenting. We are grateful to
these couples for obliging us to be far more vigilant about examining all
of our own gender-specific assumptions, specifically those that we hold
in relation to infertility.

> Alice and Edward reported that they just learned that Alice would
> be unable to carry a pregnancy to term. Although the clinician who
> worked with this couple had initially assumed that because Alice
> was a woman she would be more grief-stricken than her husband, a
> member of the clinician's team questioned that assumption. It was
> suggested that the question "Which one of you will feel saddest
> about not having the opportunity to experience a pregnancy?" be
> put to the couple. Edward said, "I think I will. . . . I've always
> wanted to see and feel our baby grow inside Alice. . . . I've been fas-
> cinated with our friends' pregnancies. I think it's such a miraculous
> process." For her part, Alice said, "I hate to say this, even though I
> want a child more than anything else in the world. If we have to
> have a baby without my experiencing pregnancy and childbirth, I'd
> feel just fine about it. . . . I've always hated any kind of physical
> inconvenience and pain, and blood terrifies me. I could easily do

without it. . . . He's the one who's always been excited about pregnancy and being there to see the baby born."

Toward the end of therapy, Alice and Edward told the clinician that gender-free questions were a very crucial part of the process for them. These questions had an important effect on each of them and on the relationship. They said this allowed each to feel comfortable with their atypical attitudes, and furthermore, it helped each to accept the other's ideas and feelings without assuming they were in any way abnormal.

Children and Parenting

A core set of beliefs evoked by the infertility experience concerns the meaning and value partners place on children and parenting. Unlike most couples, who are never confronted with infertility, those who encounter infertility are likely to think carefully and deliberately about why they want to be parents and what children mean to them.

> Lenny had, in the past, been downsized by his employer. He said that when he lost his job he was forced, for the first time in his life, to look at what working and a career meant to him, and how he saw work in relation to the other areas in his life that he valued. "It was the kind of eye-opener that I think only comes when you're knocked down," he said, "and infertility's the same kind of thing. . . . I really had to think about what it meant to be a parent, why I wanted kids. . . . It's like when I lost my job, I think I ended up being in a much better place. . . . I know that because of this [the infertility] when we get to be parents—no matter how that comes about—we're going to know why we're doing this. . . . I even think we're going to appreciate what we have more than other parents do."

For couples who are in the Dawning, Mobilization, and early Immersion phases of diagnosis and treatments, the capacity to focus on notions such as the value of children and parenting may seem less germane than it will later. Couples in later Immersion and Resolution who have faced many disappointments and failures, and have begun to think about ending medical treatment, are far more likely to reflect on what matters most insofar as children and parenting are concerned. However, no matter what the phase, it is always worthwhile to encourage the couple to explore the meaning and value they place on children and parenting. Furthermore, because these ideas may change over time, it is useful to revisit the subject periodically throughout the course of treatment.

Any discussion of the value and meaning of children and parenting ought also to include beliefs in regard to genetic relationship, adoption, and life without children. Because the chances of having a genetic relationship to the child may decline over time, it is especially important to revisit the options of adoption and no children.

Some clinicians are fearful of raising the topics of adoption or life without children, especially when they themselves see these choices as inferior, if not totally unacceptable. In this light, as one clinician told us, "I feel like I'm being defeatist and bringing up a hurtful topic." Although leaping to questions such as "What do you think about adoption?" or "What are your thoughts about not having children?" is certainly jarring and might be interpreted as callous, there are respectful ways of asking these "what if" questions and sequencing them so that the transition to these topics is less startling and harsh. The following example questions allow the clinician to cover the territory. As with other lists of questions in this text, it is fairly exhaustive and not all questions need to be asked.

- What are (were) your ideas about being a mother/father? About parenting together?
- What do you see as the value of children?
- What aspects of parenting matter most to you?
- Is having a genetically related child associated with the way you see yourself as a man/woman?
- What does the genetic relationship to your child mean to you?
- What would the absence of this relationship mean to you?
- Do you see a difference in how you might parent a genetically related child versus a child who was adopted?
- How do you imagine you would see yourself if you were a parent of a child who was adopted?
- What ideas do you have about adoptive families?
- Have you ever considered what it would be like to chose to live a life without becoming a parent?
- If you had (have) only the option of adoption or a life without children, which would seem more fitting to you?

Once beliefs are stated, questions about when and how they were learned and thoughts about alternative ideas can follow:

- Where do you think you learned [this particular idea]?
- What ideas about children, parenting, adoption, and life without children did each of you bring from your families of origin?
- Do you have family members or friends who have not had chil-

dren or have adopted? What conclusions have you drawn from their experience?

The clinician will no doubt find that although there may be some nearly universal meanings that couples associate with children and parenting, each couple is also likely to have a very unique set of ideas in these areas. Many believe that couples without children are unhappy, or that those who are enjoying their lives are selfish for not raising children. For Dorothy, it was both: "I was shocked when I asked Helene [married older cousin who had no children] if she was happy, and she said, 'Oh yes, very!' Then I thought, Boy, that's a really self-indulgent way to live your life. . . . I wanted her to be miserable."

Couples may have strong personal, familial, and/or cultural preferences for passing on their genetic lineage. Others are less concerned with lineage, but are attached to the idea of having a genetically related child because they fear that other people's genes or prenatal care will result in a child born with physical, intellectual, or emotional limitations. In the process of discovering and articulating ideas about parenting and children, couples may discover that each partner holds different sets of beliefs. Although these explorations may initially generate friction and/ or distance between partners, in the long run this kind of probing is likely to help partners understand why disputes have arisen over various treatment protocols, how they might find some middle ground or resolution, and how mutually agreeable decisions may avert problems in the future.

When asked what his thoughts were about being a father, George said he wanted "to leave my mark on the future." He could imagine doing so only with a genetically related child. Because genetic linkage was so integral to his thinking about parenthood, when the couple learned that Sally could neither produce viable eggs nor carry a baby to term, he believed he could never be a father, according to his definition, and he became depressed.

Sally came from a family in which there were several relatives diagnosed with mood disorders: One of her parents and a sibling were chronically depressed, and her family often referred to their "morose and suicidal" forebears. As a child she loved visiting other people's families and said, "Anybody else's home was always cheerful compared to mine." She had few reservations about adoption; on the contrary, she preferred *not* passing along her family's genes and thereby placing a child of hers at risk for depression. However, because George became so depressed about not having a genetically related child, Sally had undergone several cycles of infertility treatments, fearing that if she did not, George's depression would

worsen and become long-term like the depressions she had witnessed in her family.

   The clinician encouraged George to think about whether there
were other ways to "leave his mark on the future," and Sally was
asked to think about whether George's sadness could be viewed as
anything other than a psychiatric problem. Sally was able to distinguish between pathology and sadness as an expression of grief.
And, although she did not experience this sadness herself, she no
longer dreaded George becoming and remaining depressed. Sally
was then able to acknowledge George's feelings and comfort him.

   After a few weeks, no longer worried about upsetting George,
Sally began to lobby for adoption by pointing out the ways in which
fathers can pass along their life experiences, not necessarily their
genetic make-up, to their children. George, for his part, began to see
the value of this kind of legacy.

Donors

When couples consider the possibility of using a donor's genetic material, the beliefs and assumptions that are called into play vary widely. In
large part, this is due not only to the uniqueness of the protocol, but its
relative newness, especially in regard to egg donation. Because research
regarding donor children, their parents, and the donors is, to coin a
phrase, still in its infancy, would-be parents and clinicians are often at a
loss as to how to think about the donor alternative.

   We believe that, for now, until a great deal more study concerning
this unusual way of creating children becomes available, clinicians can
be most helpful to the couple by underscoring the importance of taking
time to consider seriously all the ramifications, all of their thoughts and
feelings, and how they think these might play out over time. Because this
kind of probing needs to be thorough, it is helpful to be clear with couples that the clinician's intentions are neither to encourage nor to discourage them in regard to choosing the donor option, but to help them
to make the most informed choice.

   There are those for whom the donor option is totally unacceptable.
For this group, the concept of using another person's gametes feels too
strange, too difficult to place in any familiar frame of reference, and too
fraught with uncertainty to venture the risk. Shelley, who rejected the
possibility and would not consider further discussion, put it this way:

   "It's too weird to even think about. . . . The only thoughts that I
   have are, basically, you just don't mess around with nature that
   way. . . . It's asking for trouble. I could never tell my kid that this
   is how she or he came to be. It's unfair, too big a burden. . . . I'm a

> grownup, and I cringe at the thought of a donor. How would a kid feel? Look, if I'm not comfortable, there's no way the kid will be."

Although the clinician may wish to explore such sentiments further, if both partners are relatively comfortable with their remaining alternatives—adoption or life without children—it seems unnecessary to continue discussing the subject. However, there is always the likelihood that partners will differ about the donor option. If, on further exploration, partners can reach no common ground, it is important that the clinician focus on helping the couple anticipate what the ramifications of choosing or not choosing the donor option will have on their relationship and on the life of any child that is brought into their family, given their disagreement.

For some couples, the profound desire to have a child, coupled with the belief that they will be able to handle any problems that might arise, outweighs any worries they might have about how they and their children will fare. However, if their optimism stems from the belief that the difference between having a child who is genetically related to both parents and a child conceived with only one parent's genes is negligible, the clinician can encourage the couple to think about what some real differences might be. For example, the clinician might ask the couple to consider how they would handle a child's curiosity about the donor, not as an abstract source of DNA but as a person. It can also be worthwhile for the clinician to raise the kinds of questions children ask about their origins, which we have learned from the field of adoption.

In our experience, most couples who consider using donors seem to accept the idea that the donor's role involves more than the provision of DNA, and they lean toward disclosure to the child. However, there seems to be a good deal of confusion about what the "more than just genes" represents, how it will play out in their and their children's lives, and how to talk with their children about the birth story. Because the most pressing question for most couples seems to be how to handle disclosure, they often turn to us for guidance.[2]

First is the question of who "owns" the information about the

---

[2]Two of our colleagues at the Ackerman Institute have helped us to sort out our own ideas in regard to disclosure. The first, Ronny Diamond, a member of our team with many years of clinical experience in the adoption field, provides us with a perspective that allows us to understand more fully the experiences of couples who are considering the option to use a donor, or those couples who are actually raising donor-conceived children. The second colleague is Evan Imber-Black who brings her expertise in regard to family secrets (Imber-Black, 1993). Although we suggest that clinicians working with these couples refer to Imber-Black's text, and to the adoption literature listed in Chapters 13 and 14, the following discussion offers some guidelines for thinking about donors.

donor. We believe it should belong to the child because he or she has the right to know his or her genetic origins. In addition, keeping donor conception a secret can create other problems for all family members. Just as with children who are not told they are adopted, the donor-conceived child may sense that something is not quite right and can too easily internalize this "not rightness," feeling the problem must lie with him- or herself. If and when the child learns about his or her origins later, in addition to being suddenly confronted with this powerful information, he or she must also deal with the sense of being betrayed by the parents because they kept this important fact a secret.

Second, in order for parents to talk with the child about the donor's role in the child's birth story, the parents must be comfortable with their decision to use donor gametes. In a sense, each partner's comfort with talking to the child about the birth story reflects how well each has dealt with problematic beliefs that have arisen in regard to the infertility and the losses related to not having a child genetically related to both. Therefore, if one or both partners show apprehension about talking with the child, the clinician may wish to explore this further. To initiate such discussion, the therapist can ask each partner about his or her worries in regard to telling the child about the birth story.

> Ann and Bruce were considering using a donor and surrogate. When asked about how they intended to handle this information with the child, Ann talked about the life she had led prior to her marriage. "I made really bad choices when it came to men. . . . I paid the price. I ended up with this [infertility caused by STDs]." When she imagined telling the donor child about the circumstances of his or her birth she was overwhelmed with feelings of sadness and shame: "I feel like I've brought this on my child, really let the child down."
>
> The focus of therapy shifted to her shame, sorrow, and regret about the past. With Bruce's understanding and support, she was able to be more accepting of her past and, as a result, felt less worried about disclosure. As it turned out, the couple adopted a child. "Once I felt I didn't need to prove anything and I didn't owe this to Bruce, I realized that I didn't need to go to these lengths [donor and surrogate] to be a wife and a mother."

Discomfort with disclosure can lead couples to decide to keep the information a secret. Although Ann and Bruce had planned to tell any child conceived with a donor's gametes about his or her birth story, no matter how painful they thought it would be, in the following example, the husband was so uncomfortable with disclosure that he insisted on keeping the donor information a secret. When the notion of secrecy takes on such prominence, it can be useful to explore how matters of secrecy were handled in each partner's family of origin.

> After sensing that the husband, Jim, was adamant about keeping the donor information a secret, the clinician asked the couple to talk about how issues of privacy and secrecy were handled by their respective families. As it turned out, Jim's paternal grandfather was born out of wedlock. In addition, his grandmother married while pregnant, but she did not marry the father of the child. In the small Midwestern farming town, everyone knew the identity of the genetically related father, but the subject was never discussed openly in his family.
>
> In the sessions that followed, Jim was not only able to understand how he had automatically assumed his family's habit of keeping things secret, especially secrets in relation to a child's birth story, but with the help of the clinician and the support of his wife, he stepped back and thought more about this strategy. He came to the conclusion that it had not been successful—everyone in his family seemed to know there was a secret even when they were not sure exactly what that was. And, more significantly for Jim, that atmosphere of secrecy had created problems of its own: "I always sensed something was wrong but could never quite put my finger on it. . . . If there was ever something that I felt any confusion or guilt about, anything that made me feel shame, I could never go to either of my parents. I learned early in my life you bury, you handle on your own, you don't upset other people with it." Jim came to understand that if he were to chose secrecy, he would be imposing a similar veil of confusion and shame over his child's life.

FACILITATING MOURNING

Loss is the leitmotif of the couple's encounter with infertility, and the kinds of losses are both tangible (e.g., failed medical protocols, miscarriages, still births, etc.) and intangible (e.g., experiencing a trouble-free pregnancy, having a genetically related child, as well as the anticipatory loss of not knowing whether they will ever have children [Sandelowski, 1993; see also Chapter 3, this volume]).

The clinician's awareness of and comfort with themes of loss is a crucial prerequisite to working with this population. This said, we as clinicians must bear in mind that although loss is a fundamental aspect of the human condition, not merely a central experience of infertility, we are living in a culture that has difficulty dealing with issues of loss and mourning. Not only couples, but clinicians as well may have difficulty talking about and grieving losses.

The pervasive sadness in relation to the losses of infertility is typically cumulative. Although the grief in response to early diagnoses is sometimes acute, there is often a gradual, step-by-step grieving process, starting with feeling "This is not going to be easy." This shifts to "There's a strong possibility we will not have our own [genetically related] baby," and may culminate with "There may be no child at all."

By attending to the motif of loss, the clinician can help the couple identify and address their losses. At times, this may mean probing for the implicit loss. When couples talk about, for example, not qualifying for or experiencing failure in regard to a treatment protocol, questions not only about loss but the nature of the loss need to be asked. This means stepping beyond the "How did it make you feel" level of clinical inquiry and asking about the perceived losses, for example, "What were you each hoping for?" "What did the [treatment failure, miscarriage, afternoon in the park without children, etc.] mean to you?" or "How was this one different than other losses you've encountered?"

Couples may have trouble finding words for their grief, or they may be quite eloquent in their replies. In general, we have found that questions about loss will lead to profoundly moving clinical moments. These are critical junctures, and we caution the clinician about prematurely focusing on hopeful possibilities in the future such as "You can always try again," or "Someday you'll have your baby to wheel around the park." Rather, the therapeutic goal is allowing and, if necessary, encouraging partners to express their sadness with each other and offer comfort. Although having a baby is their goal, our explicit agenda is the protection and enhancement of the couple's relationship.

We have found that partners' ability to comfort each other about their losses improves over time. At first, many are awkward about expressing sadness in front of and/or receiving comfort from the other. This is especially so when infertility produces the first serious losses the couple has yet encountered. Clinicians can approach this in a variety of ways. For example, each partner might be asked what he or she feels would be most comforting. For some, it may mean exploring beliefs associated with the expression of sadness, for example, assumptions about masculinity and stoicism. For others, a ritual may be an appropriate form of mourning.

Mourning Rituals

There are no rituals (funerals, memorial services, wakes, sitting shiva, etc.) for grieving the losses of infertility. Because these rituals facilitate the mourning process, we introduce the idea that couples can create rituals of their own. Most couples need some guidance in order to create a ritual that incorporates elements that address their losses. In suggesting and helping the couple plan a ritual, the clinician needs both to respect what the partners feel lies within their zone of comfort and to encourage them enough to inspire them to take the risk of trying something unusual. In our experience, we found that a couple is more likely to feel that creating a ritual sounds "too hokey" when the clinician has spent too little time in helping the couple articulate their loss. If treated with the importance and the solemnity it merits, the rationale for a mourning ritual makes emotional sense. Some couples arrive at inventive ways of mourning together without actually realizing they have created a mourning ritual.

> One couple had a "Bed and Chocolate Ritual." When the woman got her period after an insemination, they would both come home from work and cuddle in bed with chocolate and a video. This helped them get through another failed attempt.

Couples may prefer to mark their losses with an in-session ritual, especially if the clinician has understood their sadness and not shied away from their pain. In these instances, he or she is a respectful mourner who amplifies the solemnity of the ritual. Other couples prefer to perform their mourning ritual alone, although a discussion about how it will be executed may take place in the session. In these instances, the discussion of the ritual is likely to activate or intensify the process of mourning (see the Requiem for a Small Bubak, Chapter 14).

Mourning and Attachment

Couples struggling with infertility have typically assumed that a part of their mission in life included the creation of children, and that their roles and identity would, in large part, be defined by parenthood. Grief, therefore, is not just about the loss of the imagined child, but the loss of their unifying mission as parents, the loss of a special kind of bond: "I feel a profound sense of loss that we are not actually, physically going to be able to make love and make a baby and that we're not going to have this creature that our blood commingled in, our DNA commingled in. You know, I feel like somehow life cheated me out of something that I really, really wanted."

While we identify this loss as one of the many to mourn, we would also like to add that in the creation of and participation in mourning rituals, partners can construct different kinds of attachments with each other. These empathic bonds can have special significance and utility. Although they may not replace the unique union of parenthood, an intimate connection brought about through shared mourning is vital in helping couples weather the anguish and sorrow of infertility. When this opportunity is missed, the effects on the couple's relationship may be grievous.

> Leslie and Donald were seen after long years of what they called a "nonmarried kind of marriage." They connected their gradual disaffection not only to the infertility, but to the fact that Leslie mourned alone, at the time the infertility was diagnosed, after each treatment failure, and at various times throughout the years when feelings related to her losses were triggered.
>
> Each time Leslie pulled away from Donald to keep her mourning private, she stepped further and further away from the marriage. Donald was aware of her episodic melancholy and suspected that it stemmed from the infertility. However, he took her increasing distance as a signal that she did not want him to comfort her. Because he felt responsible for having urged her to end medical interventions, he was afraid that if he tried to step across the invisible wall she erected and console her, she might use the occasion as an opportunity to reproach him.

The Couple and the Support System: Dealing with Families and Friends

Part of understanding the effects of infertility on couples' lives is recognizing how relationships with families and friends can be altered. Because infertility makes it impossible for couples to move into the parenting phase of the life cycle, relationships with family members can be painful reminders of their situation. Although some families or individual family members can be enormously supportive, many are likely to have limited understanding of the couple's plight. Moreover, spending time with other families with children can be painful. Furthermore, if one partner finds solace in time spent with family and the other cannot tolerate family gatherings, conflicts may arise.

To address the issue of family and friends, we work with couples to find strategies for developing workable relationships during their ordeal with infertility. These vary from couple to couple. Some may look at the kinds of boundaries that existed before the infertility and evaluate whether these are still comfortable or whether a recalibration of private versus social life makes more sense now. Other couples may want to alert family members to their "temporary crisis." As one couple said,

"After our difficulties have been resolved, we will return to our normal programming."

> Carolyn was encouraged to discuss her situation with her sister, Jenny, rather than avoid her or feel resentful toward her for insisting she attend family gatherings. Carolyn reported back that she had told Jenny, "For now anyway, it's hard to attend every birthday party and dinner like we did before. It's just too hard to see [nieces and nephews] and feel sadder about not having my own children. . . . Once this period in my life is over—maybe we'll have a baby, maybe adopt one—I'll be back. It's only . . . just temporary. . . . If you can, would you please bear with me?" Although Jenny was disappointed, she understood, and she agreed to respect the "for now" terms.

Sometimes we work with couples in reaching a balance between attending and avoiding family functions so that each partner's needs are respected.

> Ed was very close to his father, whereas his wife, Alice, found her mother-in-law's attitude "ignorant and intrusive" insofar as the infertility was concerned. They reached a middle ground in that they were more selective in picking which family gatherings to attend.

It is often the case that relationships with significant family members are reconfigured as a result of the infertility. Clinicians can be helpful in resolving the tensions that develop with a parent or sibling. Generally, long-standing and unresolved conflicts tend to be rekindled by the infertility. This is another facet of the "plow of infertility": Relational problems with parents and siblings that were not addressed in the past are likely to resurface with greater intensity during this time: "If I go [to her niece's first birthday] and can't get out of my depression, my sister will accuse me of raining on her parade." Often a good indicator that some work is required is if the client reveals that he or she has cut off relations with such a family member as a result of the infertility. The clinician can offer couples the opportunity to rethink, redefine, and rework these relationships.

Another way of addressing the need for different kinds of connections to others during the ordeal of infertility is to ask couples whether there are friends and family with whom they had not spent time in the past, but who might be better company now that they are immersed in the infertility. Couples may find that they prefer to socialize with friends and family members without children, or those who are especially understanding about the infertility.

Who Knows What

It is important to help couples consider the issue of openness, privacy, or secrecy in terms of sharing information about their ordeal, and how their choices will affect their future lives and the lives of their children. Some information is especially significant and needs to be considered before sharing it with others. This includes the details regarding who is the carrier of the infertility factor, the exact medical diagnosis, and the kinds of treatment choices they are considering. We remind couples that, as difficult as it may be to remember now, there will be a future life after the infertility. Once information is disseminated, it cannot be retracted. For example, if couples share the fact that one partner is sterile and, later, the woman becomes pregnant, friends and family will know that donor gametes have been used. Although this may be perfectly acceptable to them later on, they are not in the best position to assess this now.

Clinicians treating couples during the ordeal of infertility have an opportunity to circumvent the often distressing impact of this life event. While this chapter gives an overview of our therapeutic approach, the following chapters will describe the phases of infertility and suggest specific applications of these treatment principles.

3

_⊗_

COUPLE ISSUES IN THE DAWNING PHASE

"I started to have this feeling that something wasn't right . . . getting pregnant shouldn't take this long."

CHARACTERISTICS OF DAWNING

In the early hours of the morning, one senses a barely perceptible yet gradually increasing light. Then, at some intangible moment, long before the sun is visible, one realizes that a new day has begun. Likewise, the Dawning phase of infertility is characterized by a gradual awareness that there seems to be some difficulty achieving pregnancy. This awareness grows until finally it coalesces into a certainty that action must be taken.

Typically, individuals have spent many years avoiding pregnancy, and the routine practice of contraception serves as a ritual that reinforces the presumption of fertility. In addition, if women have had abortions or men's former sexual partners became pregnant, fertility seems assured. Thus, many couples begin the process of baby making with the enthusiastic certainty that the desired event will quickly ensue. However, as the months go by and conception does not occur, the partners may begin to wonder if there is a problem.

> After 6 months of unprotected sex, Elaine and Jerry consulted a gynecologist. Following a physical exam, the physician saw no

apparent problems and reassured the couple that they would be successful, that they simply had not given the process long enough.
Elaine had had an abortion while in high school and believed she
had subsequently had two spontaneous miscarriages while in college. Jerry's previous girlfriend had become pregnant and had an
abortion while they were living together. Elaine and Jerry believed
they were "dangerously fertile" and had been scrupulous about
using birth control before they were ready to start their family.
However, after 6 more months of trying, Jerry and Elaine were
tested for infertility at the physician's suggestion. They were
stunned to learn that Jerry had so few sperm that he could be considered sterile.

In contrast, some couples may experience fears about infertility
from the beginning, prompted by the media's current focus on the condition (Faludi, 1991). Accounts of high-tech medical treatments, dramatic
stories about distraught couples who struggle with infertility, and sensational tales about donors and surrogates make good copy. Infertility
seems to have been added to the growing list of diseases, disorders, and
dysfunctions presented by the media as modern-day plagues. Therefore,
it is not surprising that there are couples with relatively few risk factors
for infertility (couples who are young and healthy) who, after their first
unsuccessful attempts to become pregnant, begin to suspect that they
may be infertile.

Many older couples who have postponed childbearing are also concerned about infertility, and they often have some awareness that the
longer they wait to get pregnant, the more they may compromise their
fertility (see Chapter 1 and the Appendix). They have been exposed to
media coverage for more years than younger couples and are likely to
have contemporaries who are struggling with infertility. Witnessing others' distress and imagining the profound effect infertility would have on
their own lives, older couples may be quick to assume that they too are
infertile.

Some men and women approach childbearing knowing they have
preexisting medical conditions that may interfere with or prevent conception (e.g., women diagnosed with endometriosis are usually told that
the condition will affect their fertility). However, the yearning for a
genetically related child can lead people to deny or downplay their biological limitations. For example, they may hold out hope that an error
was made by the physician who first diagnosed their condition or that
their impediment is less severe than originally thought. Some even hope
that their condition has magically cured itself. For these individuals, it
may take repeated failures at trying to become pregnant for them to be
convinced that there is indeed a physiological impairment.

Candace could not accept her infertility until she had seen the lab results and heard the physician's confirmation: "It was like when my father died. I knew it was coming; the doctors told us just how long he had to live, and I thought I was preparing myself. But it was only at his death that it hit me: I'd never see him again. It felt that way when Dr. Chen [the infertility specialist] showed me the test results. I knew about my condition—the doctors told me when I was 19—but seeing the lab report was like reading a death certificate."

Couples may assiduously avoid facing the specter of infertility, thus preventing awareness of a possible problem from emerging. Some women in their 40s may be unconcerned about their chances of getting pregnant, even if they have been having unprotected sex for months without conceiving. They may entertain the fantasy that because they look young and healthy, their eggs are as fertile as those of a younger woman.

Rosemary, age 47, went to several infertility specialists looking for a doctor who would treat her. "Everyone tells me I look 10 years younger than my age," she said. "I just assumed my eggs were like those of a 37-year-old woman."

THE CRISIS AND TRAUMA OF INFERTILITY

For the most part, couples in the Dawning phase do not experience infertility as a traumatic crisis. However, for those who are inclined to a catastrophic world view, the anguish that is the hallmark of later phases may arise even at this early date.

Dawning Awareness

Many couples fully expect to be able to get pregnant once they make the decision to do so (Abbey et al., 1992; Greil, 1991; Mahlstedt, 1985; Miall, 1987; Veevers, 1980). The dawning awareness emerges slowly, accompanied by a moderate concern. If they have no history of infertility or medical problems, and if they are under 40, they presume that conception will occur with no difficulty. But after a few months of trying with no results, one of the partners will realize that it is not going as he or she expected. The woman, more often than not, will begin to wonder, "Didn't we make love when I was ovulating? Why am I getting my period?" Some people may begin to worry after only 2 months, whereas others, in spite of the media's coverage of infertility, may not have any

inkling of a problem for months or even years. But, eventually, they realize that it is not happening as easily as expected. Couples may rational-
ize why it might be taking so long to conceive, concluding, for example,
that their attempts did not coincide with ovulation. Some may turn to
books and start charting their temperature or begin using over-the-
counter ovulation detection kits.

Anticipatory Loss

As the awareness dawns, couples face the prospect that getting pregnant
may be more difficult than they expected. Although they realize that it
will be inconvenient and costly, and take greater effort on their part,
they rarely consider the idea that it will not happen.

But some, particularly those who have paid close attention to stories about infertility in the media and who have a predisposition to
thinking the worst, may react more strongly to the failure to conceive.
They begin to imagine that they might never have a child, thus anticipating a loss that may never occur (Sandelowski, 1993). Their longing
makes them particularly aware of parenting in their surroundings. Suddenly it seems to them as if everyone is pregnant or pushing a baby car-
riage. Even seeing parents with older children can be painful and prompt
grief over the idea that they might never have that experience.

IMPACT ON THE COUPLE RELATIONSHIP

As discussed earlier, partners often cycle through the various stages of
the infertility experience at different times. When they are out of synch it
can lead to tension and conflict in the relationship. Other areas of conflict include differing styles of coping and gender differences.

Coping Styles

Differences between partners can quickly emerge over whether there is
any reason to be concerned about getting pregnant. People may also get
upset with the ways in which their partners are handling their anxiety. A
partner with a more optimistic disposition, for example, may remain relatively untroubled until infertility has been confirmed, while his or her
partner may be very worried. When the anxiety of one partner is not
shared by the other, the dynamic balance between worry and reassurance can tip. Polarizations may escalate (Greil, 1991; Mahlstedt, 1985)
as the worrier's alarm leads the optimistic partner to reassure him or her
so much that the worrier becomes more apprehensive. Unintentionally,

the comforter encourages the worrier to worry more, and the worrier induces the comforter to reassure still more forcefully.

"When Frank kept saying, 'You're getting upset over nothing,' I got really upset," said Cheryl. "I felt like I was alone in this. . . . I was not only going to have to deal with infertility, but he was going to fight it all the way."

"I looked at Cheryl and said to myself, 'She is really acting screwy about this,' " said Frank. "She never seemed this way before . . . something must be going on, you know, some kind of panic thing. I figured the best I could do was to calm her down." The more Frank tried to calm Cheryl, the more upset she became. By the time she spoke to her gynecologist, she was so distraught that the doctor thought Cheryl was indeed having some kind of emotional breakdown and suggested she take a vacation.

"When I insisted he begin testing me, you know, doing some kind of workup, he gave me this big smile and handed me a slip of paper. I looked down and saw it wasn't any referral for a test, it was a prescription for Xanax! On the way home I wondered if I was acting a little kooky, and even found some reassurance in thinking I might be. Then it would be possible that I was not infertile. I was just nuts. When Frank asked me how it went, I felt trapped between two people who wouldn't hear me. . . . I knew if I told him the doctor agreed with him, I would lose my only ally . . . but I couldn't lie to Frank . . . and of course Frank gloated when I told him what the doctor said. I wanted to kill him."

Cheryl's fears did not abate. The comprehensive workup confirmed what Cheryl had feared: She was unable to conceive. "It was a sad victory," she said, "who wants to be right about this!"

GENDER DIFFERENCES: WHY WOMEN WORRY SOONER

For a variety of reasons, women are likely to be the first to sound the infertility alarm (Abbey et al., 1992; Meyers et al., 1995a). First, their interest in pregnancy is often greater than their husbands' because although there have been cultural changes regarding the role of women and many women no longer define themselves solely as mothers, there is still greater emphasis placed on motherhood than on fatherhood. Second, whereas a man's fertility depends almost exclusively on the quantity and quality of his sperm, a woman's fertility is multifaceted. Her ovaries must produce an egg, her follicles must successfully transport the egg to the site of fertilization, her body must produce a chemically compatible fluid to receive the sperm, and her uterus must provide an adequate environment for the fertilized ovum to implant and the fetus to develop. Many women today know that there can be a variety of problems. Third, magazines designed for female audiences are far more likely to contain articles about reproduction and children than are magazines geared to a male readership. Because stories about infertility and its treatments are often featured, motherhood and the possibility of infertility are increasingly linked. Lastly, the themes of pregnancy and childbirth are more likely to arise in women's conversations with each other than in men's conversations.

SECONDARY INFERTILITY

Secondary infertility, which by definition occurs after couples have been able to conceive and bear children, presents with a different face. Unless the woman is of advanced maternal age, or there is reason to suspect that a couple's fertility has been jeopardized in some other way, prior conceptions, pregnancies, and deliveries provide convincing proof that the couple can have children. Assuming they are fertile, some couples with secondary infertility may ignore or deny the signs of failure and wait longer before consulting a physician than couples who never had children: "For a long time we assumed that we were just not getting the timing right . . . maybe my ovulation cycle was not so predictable. . . . Then we realized this is really taking a long time. What could it be?"

Others quickly realize that, compared to earlier successes getting pregnant, something is wrong. These couples consult their physicians after relatively few attempts to conceive: "I knew something wasn't right almost immediately—the first time I got pregnant on the first try."

4

THERAPEUTIC APPROACH
IN THE DAWNING PHASE

"I look at the world, the world of parents and children,
and I feel like a hungry child staring through the
window of a restaurant and seeing all these happy
families inside having a good time."

In the Dawning phase, it is unusual to see couples for infertility-related problems. Nevertheless, we have included several treatment strategies that may also be implemented later as the need for them arises.

PRESENTING PROBLEM

Although during the Dawning phase couples are unlikely to seek therapy for concerns related solely to infertility, some couples may be in therapy when their difficulties getting pregnant first arise. If they have postponed having children because of their concerns about the relationship, when things improve they may decide to begin their families. Then, if they encounter problems getting pregnant, the therapist may witness the dawning process as one or both partners gradually realize that something is amiss.

Some couples in this phase may present regarding ambivalence about the relationship or the decision to have children.

Susan and Steve, a young couple in their 20s, were not married at the time they entered therapy. Susan had been diagnosed with endometriosis, and the doctor had encouraged her to conceive as soon as possible. However, Steve was ambivalent about the relationship and was particularly focused on his doubts about whether he wanted Susan to be the mother of his children.

Childless couples, especially those who are approaching the end of their childbearing years, may come to a therapist in order to clarify their feelings about whether or not to have children. They may wonder whether they can strengthen the relationship before entering the parenting stage of their lives, or they may want to come to terms with a decision not to have children. They may even consider ending the relationship in order to find other partners with whom to raise children. However, the "baby agenda" is not always explicit.

Even when couples state that the question of children is the catalyst that brought them to therapy, resolving their difficulties and/or improving the couple relationship can take time. During this interval, couples may or may not realize that the risk of infertility is increasing. Unfortunately, the following is an increasingly common situation:

Amy had no children, and Mike had children from a previous marriage. They agreed at the time of their marriage not to have children, but over time, Amy began to feel otherwise. Mike remained firm about their original agreement, and they came for treatment because of their impasse. In therapy, Mike came to the realization that if he continued to refuse, he could lose his wife or she might come to resent him for denying her this experience, so, after an extended time, he agreed to have a child. However, they had delayed so long that when they began trying, Amy was diagnosed with infertility due to her age. Mike felt remorse because had he not objected, she might have had a child.

Although some couples recognize the risk in delaying childbearing, they may assume that with the help of medicine they can overcome any difficulties that arise. In such cases, the dawning process is the clinician's, not the couple's, in that he or she may be more concerned about the possibility of infertility than the clients are.

Having a first child is a life-cycle decision that calls the relationship into bold relief (Carter & McGoldrick, 1989). Unlike engagement and marriage, which are often perceived as less than permanent in this age of no-fault divorce, having children is seen as a long-term commitment. If couples encounter difficulties trying to get pregnant, one or both partners may realize they do not want to continue the relationship, whereas if they had gotten pregnant right away, they might have stayed married.

For couples who experienced primary infertility but were able to have a child, the question of having a second child may be fraught with more conflict, as it involves reentering the medical arena with all the emotional, physical and financial upheaval that this involves. In this situation, couples may enter therapy to try to resolve their differences about how to proceed.

RESPECT AND LIMIT THE IMPACT OF THE INFERTILITY

When worries about infertility arise, it is important to treat them seriously. The therapist's response should be neither overly alarmed nor falsely reassuring. Similar to the advice of family and friends, clinicians often attempt to normalize fears with statements such as "I'm sure you don't have anything to worry about—you'll get pregnant." Although a therapist's desire to comfort a worried couple may arise out of the best of intentions, he or she cannot be sure of their fertility. In addition, blanket reassurances subtly reinforce the myth that failure to achieve a pregnancy is associated with too much anxiety. For example, if a woman raises the concern, the clinician's reassurance may feel patronizing. Furthermore, if her partner has taken a placating posture, the woman may feel outnumbered; she may stop talking about her worries but feel them even more deeply. And, if one partner—most often the man—has been less inclined to voice concern about the possibility of infertility, he or she may take a cue from the therapist and try to push his own fears away. As a result, the partners are unable to share their mutual worries.

One way to offer support while at the same time allowing partners to air their worries might be as follows: "Until you can be more certain, it does seem hard not to worry," or "Although many couples feel the same way, if you're this worried about it, you might want to check it out with your gynecologist." Later, rather than leaving the impression that infertility is just a medical matter and that couples should restrict their worries to their physician's office, it is helpful to follow up on the medical consultation and then discuss the medical *and* emotional picture.

THE THERAPIST'S ROLE

When is it appropriate for a therapist to broach the subject of infertility? Although the Society for Assisted Reproductive Technology (SART;

1998) recommends telling patients the facts about infertility, therapists may feel that it is too intrusive to discuss reproductive issues and may therefore avoid initiating such discussions. Just as partners engage in protective behavior, shielding one another from any negative thoughts each may have about the other (see Chapter 7 for a detailed discussion of this issue), so too do clinicians have the urge to protect the couple.

In this case, supervision, working with a team, or case consultation can be extremely helpful in identifying any blind spots or biases the clinician may have about raising sensitive issues with a couple. It is important to probe the issue or ask permission to discuss infertility, saying, for example, "Do you think you might want children some time in the future?", as couples often benefit from talking about topics they have avoided. By initiating these difficult discussions, the therapist helps the partners to clarify their positions and attitudes regarding childbearing, the relationship, sexuality, identity, and treatment decisions. Although at times it was uncomfortable to do, we increasingly realized that asking the difficult questions was of great benefit to the clients. As one woman said: "You asked questions that other people would . . . feel maybe were too intrusive, questions that were really specific about the infertility and really probing. . . . You asked us questions that nobody ever asks us."

If the clinician raises the possibility of infertility, he or she must guard against infusing the discussion with an urgency that the couple may not feel. The therapist may concur with the cultural assumption, discussed below, that everyone wants children, and this belief may color his or her stance when raising the issue of when the couple plans to start a family.

LOCATE THE COUPLE ON THE TRAJECTORY

In the Dawning phase, it is helpful for the clinician to realize that the couple is on the threshold of what may be a long medical and emotional trek, and that their trajectory will include a relatively predictable sequence of events. The therapist can help the couple cope with the current stresses by telling them that many of the problems they have begun to experience are not unusual when couples start to confront the prospect of infertility.

EXPLORE COUPLES' BELIEF SYSTEMS

The statistical risks of infertility for women between the ages of 35 and 40 (see Chapter 1) are often higher than couples realize. Thus, it is not surprising to find that many couples believe there is little cause for concern until the woman reaches 40.

> Nat and Sarah were shocked when Sarah encountered serious infertility problems at age 37. They were both upset that their previous therapist hadn't raised the issue of children or the risks of infertility. They said that if he had, they would have made the decision to get pregnant while continuing to work on their difficulties: "We probably would've had more reason to work things out, not keep our arguments going, if we knew the clock was running out. . . . We thought we had a lot of time."

It must be stressed that the clinician's introduction of important topics, such as children and infertility, may produce repercussions within the couple, and between the couple and the therapist. Clients may react angrily and question the therapist's right to intrude. Clinicians must use their discretion regarding the timing of the questioning. There are situations in which exploration of such topics may not only put undue burden on the couple's relationship, but may even prove to be countertherapeutic. For example, if couples are in extreme distress, and/ or if they are unable to resolve major differences, it would be premature to raise the larger issues of children and fertility. When the clinician determines that a conversation about children seems appropriate, it is important to encourage the couple to discuss all options including genetically related and adopted children, as well as the option of not having children.

This means giving equal time to exploration of childfree living, as this is often invested with negative connotations. Our culture assumes that couples "naturally" want to have children (Greil, 1991; Hendricks, 1985; Miall, 1987; Veevers, 1980); therefore, normalizing less culturally acceptable feelings (the trials of childrearing and the pleasures of a life without children) can be both liberating and guilt reducing. People may believe that they are not suited to be parents because they have doubts about the responsibilities of parenting and enjoy their lives without children. On the other hand, if they are leaning toward a life without children, they may need an opportunity to talk about the sadness associated with relinquishing the possibility of having children, as well as their concerns about the social stigma they may encounter.

Discussions about children may evoke different responses from each partner and are likely to follow gender lines. In general, women are more invested in parenting than men are. However, although the awareness of these differences has its value, listening for exceptions to gender stereotypes is equally, if not more, important. An accepting attitude on the part of the clinician also models how partners might listen to each other's thoughts and feelings.

The following list of questions may help to initiate discussions between partners regarding children and infertility, topics that may have been ignored or avoided by the couple.

- Have the two of you thought about if and when you want to have children?
- Have you always assumed that having children was not a matter of choice?
- As you are both interested in having children, when are you planning to get pregnant?
- Are either of you concerned about the possibility of infertility?
- Do either of you have any special medical conditions that cause you to worry about infertility?
- What do you know about how a woman's age relates to infertility?
- Have you discussed any of this with your gynecologist? What has he or she said?
- Would you prefer to work out all your relational difficulties before having children, even if it puts your fertility at risk? Or, would you rather risk having difficulties in your relationship, but have children?

Regarding a life without children:

- If you chose not to have children, how do you imagine it will affect your relationships with your family and friends?
- Which one of you might have the harder time not having children? Which one of you might have the harder time having children?
- If there are differences between you about these matters, how do you think you will resolve them?

When couples want to have children, but plan to start their families after a woman's 35th birthday, the clinician is presented with the option of raising or not raising the connection between a woman's age and the decline of fertility. It can be useful to ask the couple if they are aware of this connection and if they are interested in including this information in the therapeutic conversation. When couples opt to do so, the therapist needs to communicate the idea that he or she does not intend to influence their decision about whether and when to have children, but to help them make the most informed choices.

Broach the Meaning and Value
of Children and Parenting

As mentioned in Chapter 2, as couples become aware of the possibility that they may have to deal with infertility problems, they may also become acutely aware of the meaning that having children holds for them (Mathews, 1991; Mathews & Mathews, 1986). For some, this will be the first time their beliefs and feelings about children are made explicit to both themselves and their partners. Some partners may discover that they have similar attitudes about children: "We realized for the first time that kids were very important to each of us, maybe even at the heart of our marriage."

Other couples may discover their differences: "We both wanted children, but he wanted them much more than me." If left unresolved, these submerged differences often lead to conflict during the later phases of infertility. For example, subsequent disagreements about medical options often mirror unresolved differences about how much value each partner places on having genetically related children.

In addition to the questions about the meaning and value of children listed in Chapter 2, it is also useful to find out which attitudes toward parenting the partners have adopted from their particular families of origin and which from society, and whether they believe that being a parent confers a special, perhaps adult status, and that adulthood is defined by parenthood.

- Are there unresolved issues related to your family of origin, legacies from your own childhood that affect your wish to have children?
- Is having a child a means of attaining status in your families and in society?

Later, in the Immersion phase, couples often feel an intense need to get pregnant at all cost. The assumption that pregnancy is a necessity may need to be revisited at that time. Therefore, discussions about parenting, children, and genetic relatedness can be initiated during the Dawning phase. The underlying beliefs that drive the desire for children are often covert, or if stated, are expressed in general statements such as "Having children was why we were put on this planet." Examining these ideas more closely is useful in helping couples understand not only what they feel about having children, but why they feel as they do. In such an exploration, alternatives can emerge; for example, if parenting represents a way of giving meaning to one's existence, what other ways might there be to achieve that goal? Perhaps the desire for a child is driven by legacies of the family of origin such as a death and the fantasy of a replacement child, or current issues in the family such as wanting to bring forth a child for a dying relative.

> Mary and Donald, a couple in their 20s, had been trying to conceive a baby for 6 months when Mary's mother developed cancer. Although she and Donald would not otherwise have consulted a physician or even considered themselves infertile, she began to worry that she might not have her child before her mother died. Mary wanted to give her mother the pleasure of a grandchild and fantasized that by giving her mother a joyous event to anticipate, she might prolong her mother's life. The couple consulted an infertility specialist much sooner than they would have under "normal conditions." It was then that they learned of Mary's infertility problems.

In such a case, would resolution of the family problem free the individual or couple to find another way of parenting? Clarifying such issues may help the couple to avoid some of the driven quality of the Immersion phase of infertility and also pave the way for more open communication between them when the going gets tough.

END OF DAWNING

Anita and Arnold were married for 10 years, had never practiced birth control, and had never had a pregnancy. When Anita turned 38, she and Arnold realized that her childbearing years would soon be over. At that point, they decided it was time to consult a physician.

Although couples come to it in different ways, the awareness that there may be a problem with infertility eventually occurs. Couples may assume it will be smooth sailing, especially if they are young and healthy, or have already had a child. But as the months go by with no pregnancy, the couple comes to the realization that they will have to take action, to step out of the expected order of events and go for a medical consultation.

The time span between the dawning of awareness and a consultation with a physician varies. On one end of the continuum are those who schedule appointments with their doctors after only a few months of trying to conceive. On the other end of the continuum are those who delay taking any action until they near the end of their childbearing years and/ or after a specific event precipitates the desire to have children.

5

⌘

COUPLE ISSUES IN THE MOBILIZATION PHASE

"She'd been saying, 'We've got to do something about this—look into it.' I kept saying, 'Don't push the panic button yet.' I agreed to go [for a medical opinion] just to calm her fears . . . but once the tests started coming back I realized we were facing something pretty serious."

CHARACTERISTICS OF MOBILIZATION

During Mobilization, couples shift into active gear and start to investigate medical assessment and treatment. Whether they start with a gynecologist or an infertility specialist, couples may investigate several clinics or doctors in their search for competence and comfort. If the physician sees reason to believe there may be a problem, a battery of medical tests is initiated. Although the diagnostic phase may be brief if the condition can be diagnosed quickly (e.g., low sperm count, anovulation, early menopause), it is sometimes drawn out for years (e.g., cases of reproductive tract or pelvic environment dysfunctions). Most distressing for couples is idiopathic infertility, in which no problem areas are found and yet there are repeated failures to conceive.

If biological explanations are found for the infertility during the diagnostic process, distress can be offset by the hope of successful treatment. These couples are often buoyed by the possibility of a solution; many describe an initial surge of optimism. Although they recognize that the process of getting pregnant will take longer than expected, they have reason to believe there will be light at the end of the tunnel: "I think we'll get there, but it's just going to be harder than we thought." Others may be so devastated by the possibility of not conceiving a baby that they can rally little enthusiasm for the suggested medical protocols.

During Mobilization, partners may form enduring patterns of communication with the medical system, family and friends, and each other. These patterns will affect the couple's experience in later phases. For some, this phase marks the beginning of ongoing distress, both individually—the onset of the *infertile identity*—and as a couple—communication gaps, sexual problems, and so forth.

MEDICAL PROCEDURE

As mentioned in Chapter 1, the infertility rates are 40% female factor, 40% male factor, 10% interactional, and 10% unexplained (idiopathic) (Maars, 1997). Therefore, when the couple goes for the initial evaluation, it is important that both partners be tested for infertility. Briefly, the medical procedures that a couple may encounter during the early stages of infertility treatment include ovulation testing, sperm testing, and, possibly, cervical function testing (Marrs, 1997). Tests for problems in the reproductive tract (e.g., hysterosalpingogram) and pelvic environment (e.g., laparoscopy) are more invasive and may occur later in the process of treatment. In addition to testing, the woman may receive a prescription for ovulation-stimulating drugs, which can have a variety of side effects such as intense mood swings and ovulation hyperstimulation (see the Appendix for details).

THE CRISIS AND TRAUMA OF INFERTILITY

Infertility represents a crisis, an out-of-life-cycle stage in a couple's life. Each phase of infertility reveals different aspects of this trauma.

Shock and Disbelief

When couples enter the Mobilization phase and decide to go to the doctor, they often do not expect that any indication of infertility will be found: "We worried, we were anxious and concerned, but we never actually thought they were going to find something wrong." If a diagnosis of infertility is confirmed, the couple may react with shock and disbelief. Couples may doubt the diagnosis and seek a second opinion, assuming that this will refute the first. As with the diagnosis of cancer or some other life-threatening disease, couples may bridle at the truth, denying the possibility and hoping to find out that it was all a dreadful mistake. For couples experiencing secondary infertility, the shock may be particularly severe. Having already borne a child, they are completely taken by surprise at finding that they are no longer fertile.

Another blow is to learn that something within one's own or one's partner's body is not functioning properly. This shock is exacerbated in individuals who felt they were in control of their bodies—taking vitamins, eating a nutritious diet, and so forth—and saw themselves as particularly healthy, even athletic. In such cases, the diagnosis of infertility due, for example, to a low sperm count or a malfunctioning ovary can be particularly disturbing.

Couples who have led relatively carefree lives may be stunned by a diagnosis of infertility. Having never before encountered a life-disrupting crisis, they may be unprepared for the idea that anything bad could ever happen to them. Infertility may be their first experience of life being out of their control. For people who have endured previous hardship (due to chronic illness, accident, early loss, etc.), infertility may be less of a shock. Indeed, individuals who habitually perceive the cup as being half empty may react by saying, "It figures; this always happens to me." However, in cases where a prior serious illness has contributed to the problem, people may minimize the infertility and associated losses. They are so happy to have survived their illness that the inability to have children may seem less overwhelming.

Another aspect of shock and disbelief is the feeling of "Why me?", a sense that life is unfair. Often, couples cannot understand why they are being deprived of a child when others, who do not even want children, have them easily. Clients may recall stories about women leaving their newborns to die; these couples are distressed at the perceived injustice of their own inability to have a child who would be wanted and cherished.

People may also confront their own mortality when they receive a diagnosis of infertility. As with the death of a parent, the buffer between oneself and death is removed and one feels very vulnerable. With the prospect of biological childlessness, in addition to any fear about one's own mortality, one is confronted with the possibility of leaving nothing for posterity. Whereas men tend to define themselves based on their work, for women, work is important but having children often holds equal or greater weight. Gender differences notwithstanding, men also feel shock at the idea that their genetic line will not continue, that after they die, nothing of themselves will remain.

LOSS

When diagnosed with infertility, couples may initially experience feelings of disappointment, sadness, and anger, which generally become more intense as time goes on. As with other crises, partners may blame themselves for bad choices, such as delaying childbearing, or imagined transgressions, such as having had an abortion. They may also blame their physicians for not warning them about the risks of infertility. But once couples realize that the process of having a child will be different than they had expected, they are faced with the first losses of infertility. These losses may be traumatic, and the clinician should be aware of their significance.

Loss of Control over Sex Life and Problem-Free Conception

During the Dawning phase, when couples engage in sexual intercourse with the intention of getting pregnant, their pleasure is often heightened. They are liberated from the fear of having an accidental pregnancy, a fear that usually diminishes sexual pleasure. Freed from the constraints of contraception and fear, love making can be more spontaneous, and there is a special thrill to knowing that one may be making a baby. Partners often feel closer to each other at such times, and they even describe their feelings toward each other and the world in spiritual terms: "I was really into this fantasy that we would make love and there would be this beautiful moment of conception and it would be very meaningful."

However, once infertility becomes the uninvited guest in the couple's bed, the imperative of baby making changes all that. Couples are typically required to schedule their intercourse during the fertile days of the woman's menstrual cycle, and sex becomes mechanical. The loss of spontaneity in the couple's sexual relationship can be upsetting:

> Ron and Danielle had been trying to conceive for several months when they came for therapy: "Our sex life had been fine, fine to robust I would say," Ron told us. "But when we started trying to conceive, we, I got increasingly stressed out. Not in general, but particularly on days when Danielle thought, 'By God, this is it. I'm ovulating. Let's go!' I would freak out. I would either get and lose an erection, or not get one at all, and that would create incredible tension and difficulty for us."

In addition to anxiety and uncertainty undermining the couple's sex life, their expectation of having a problem-free conception is thwarted.

Their imagined conception—a private occasion, joyously undertaken with no worries—has been lost and replaced by a battery of medical exams, office procedures, and unwelcome intrusions. This may precipitate feelings of sadness for the couple, although in the face of the hope that accompanies the Mobilization stage, this loss may not be acknowledged.

Loss of Faith in One's Body

The diagnosis of infertility may trigger a loss of confidence in one's own body, a feeling that one's accustomed trust in one's body has been disrupted. This may be exacerbated if there is any previous physical problem or disability. The idea that one must resort to medical intervention to achieve something that should be a "natural" function can feel shameful.

Loss of Privacy and Intimacy

The infertility work up requires medical examinations, questions about sexual behavior, and a technical approach to reproduction, all of which seriously compromise couples' privacy and intimacy. Many find it acutely embarrassing to discuss their sexual practices with a doctor. In addition, physical exams and diagnostic procedures may be uncomfortable, and the timetable requiring sex during the ovulatory phase makes physical intimacy feel stilted and awkward. This loss of privacy can evoke deep feelings of shame and violation.

Barrier to Achievement of Full Adult Status

Because the role of parent is central to many couples' identities, the inability to have a child means a failure to fulfill that role; one's identity, one's sense of "who I am and who I planned to be," is threatened. Furthermore, in many families, achieving full membership among the adults is determined by the birth of the first child; couples without children may be treated as children. Infertility, therefore, acts as a barrier preventing couples from assuming adult status within their families and communities:

> At a family wedding, a couple who was having difficulty conceiving was put at a table with the teenagers. "We're older than many of my cousins with children!" said the wife. "Until we produce a kid, I doubt they will see me as an adult. . . . Will they be putting us at the young-adult table until we're 60? And then what? At the old people's table!"

IMPACT ON THE COUPLE RELATIONSHIP

A "Make or Break" Experience

Many couples report that infertility can "make or break" a marriage (Rolland, 1994). Those who withstand the test make statements such as "It has made us stronger," "We learned a lot about ourselves and each other and about marriage," or "We feel if we got through this, we can get through anything." On the other hand, couples who were unable to withstand the negative impact of infertility said that their marriages were never the same afterward. One person said, "I think we both died a little, and the marriage died a lot." Another, discussing her divorce, said, "It was probably the infertility that ended the relationship."

As partners cope with the social isolation that can result from coping with infertility, their bonds with each other may be either strengthened or weakened. For those who adopt a united position, the "us-against-them" approach is likely to strengthen their ties. Alternatively, partners may blame each other for the infertility or become chronically distressed, even depressed. In this case, they may become easily irritated with and/or avoidant of each other. For example, after a family gathering in which their infertile status contributes to the distress experienced, a mutually supportive couple can often comfort each other, but a similar event may increase tensions for partners who are divided by the infertility.

Some couples are able to develop mutually satisfying coping strategies to deal with the stresses and losses of infertility. They may struggle, but they eventually arrive at what might be described as an emotional consensus that respects each partner's needs. Because this kind of consensus is the task of marriage in general, and for most couples is a difficult process even in the best of circumstances, infertility inevitably provides a "crisis" and an "opportunity" for the relationship (Johnson, 1994).

Secrecy and Protection

Couples are often reluctant to share their deepest feelings and thoughts concerning the infertility. Although this is to be expected with partners who approach all painful matters stoically or with those who have always had problems sharing disturbing thoughts and feelings with one another, infertility may also generate communication problems with previously intimate and expressive couples.

It may be that the thoughts and feelings raised by the infertility feel too threatening to share with one's partner. As mentioned earlier, individuals may, for example, start to question their own or their partner's physical desirability; have fantasies of fleeing the relationship, perhaps to find another partner; or they may worry that the other has these thoughts as well: "If I tell him what's going on inside of me, I may not want to hear what he's thinking. . . . I couldn't handle that on top of everything else." The concern about injuring the other or oneself is especially acute when partners are having difficulty sustaining their equilibrium in the face of infertility.

As the months of infertility wear on, and as infertility starts to dominate their lives, partners may turn to friends, family, or individual therapists for support. However, when conversations about the infertility and its treatments remain outside of the couple's relationship, as the pace and intensity of treatment increases, problems can arise. The partners may have very different ideas about how to proceed and about the meaning of the various options. With faulty communication, they may come to an impasse, or one may proceed without consulting the other, reserving deliberations for friends or therapists. Over time, these triangulated relationships may cause rifts and tensions between partners.

> Infertility shifted the relationship between Mia and Tom. Although the couple had always been best friends and confidants, once Tom's infertility was diagnosed and his erectile problems began, Mia began to turn more and more to her female friends and relatives. She used them as a forum in which to discuss her growing frustration with Tom and as a source of comfort and advice. Although she believed that if she discussed Tom's difficulties with him, she would only make matters worse, in the midst of handling her distress over infertility, she discovered she had lost the support of her best friend, Tom.

Gender Differences

During Mobilization, as the concern about infertility builds, gender-linked differences between partners are likely to surface. Although both partners may be distressed, compared with their husbands, wives are likely to be more troubled by the prospect of not becoming pregnant (Andrews et al., 1992; Daniluk, 1988; Freeman et al., 1985; Lalos et al., 1985; Wirtberg, 1992). This often leads to women's taking greater initiative in pursuing medical intervention, which can be attributed to differences between men's and women's identity formation and the inescapable biological fact that a woman's body is the site of conception and pregnancy. Although the gender gap between partners typically widens during Immersion, during the Mobilization phase the relationship may show the early signs of strain.

Communication Gaps

Women who talk to their partners may experience less distress (McEwan et al., 1987). However, men often feel worse after talking about the crisis, and, assuming that their partners feel the same, they may remain silent, hoping that this silence will protect their partners from further distress (Wirtberg, 1992). Because men may communicate less distress about being childless, women often conclude that men do not share the desire for a child. Unfortunately, when men appear unperturbed by treatment failures, women may feel rejected, unsupported, and/or weaker than their partners. For their part, men may be confused about how best to relate to and support their partners; they may even accept their partners' perception of them as unfeeling or less devoted to the idea of having a child (Wirtberg, 1992).

Because men are socialized to regard menstruation, reproduction, and infertility as "women's problems," men may find it difficult to talk about the infertility. The degree of intimacy required for adequate discussions regarding medical plans necessitates an alteration in the couple's relationship, one that both partners may at first find difficult.

> "In our family we never talked about these things—that is, the men [didn't]. I assume the women did, together, by themselves," said Nat. "Suddenly the doctor was talking about sexual matters that frankly made me blush. I kept wanting to disappear from the room. At those early meetings, I could barely look at her or Sarah."
>
> "I felt strange having him there too," added Sarah. "I went to all the clinic appointments by myself until the doctor said, 'Look, we really need to have your husband here.' We had to get over a lot, and now we're very different; we talk. It's too bad it took the infertility to get us here."

Coping Styles: Problem Solving
versus Expression of Emotion

Conflict often arises over differences in coping styles. A more action-oriented partner may try to push ahead with treatment or, conversely, may want to avoid treatment failures by moving straight to adoption. The other partner may prefer a slower process, with ample time and opportunity to express him- or herself. Action-oriented partners may think that talking about feelings and expressing sadness is a waste of time and, indeed, may feel worse when they talk about their pain. On a practical level, this becomes problematic if the action-oriented partner rushes into a precipitous decision that has long-term effects, not only for the other partner, but for the couple and any possible offspring as well.

On an emotional level, the different coping styles can lead to feelings of isolation and disconnection between the partners.

Although the cultural stereotypes of men and women might lead one to conclude that the action-oriented type is usually male and the partner who needs to express emotions is female, not every couple fits this mold (Nachtigall et al., 1992). Despite the fact that we have noticed a tendency for men to lean toward cognitive, action-oriented styles and for women to need their partners to listen to them and talk about the infertility, significant exceptions do occur. Interestingly, when older women feel they are waging a battle against time, they may be the ones to rush ahead regardless of their own or their partner's feelings. Equally noteworthy are instances when men experience more anguish then their partners and have a greater need to express their pain and grief.

> Ned was greatly troubled by the thought of not having a genetic heir, whereas Hilda was far more saddened by the idea of losing the chance of mothering, whether with a genetically related or an adopted child. Hilda was vexed that Ned was slowing down the adoption process because he wasn't ready to move ahead.

Sexual Relationship

Sex fosters marital intimacy, relieves tensions, and provides closeness. For some, it is a means of achieving that closeness, whereas for others it is a natural consequence of intimacy.

As discussed above, infertility can significantly disrupt a couple's sex life (Andrews et al., 1992; Berg & Wilson, 1991; Daniluk, 1988; Hirsch & Hirsch, 1989). As treatment protocols typically require sexual intercourse to take place at specific times in the woman's ovulation cycle, having to make love on demand strips the act of passion and spontaneity. These conditions can result in performance difficulties for men. Wives' resulting disappointment and frustration is, understandably, great. This is often related less to their diminished sexual pleasure than to the obstacle that performance failure presents to getting pregnant. One wife wondered if there were some conscious or unconscious motive that was driving her husband to "sabotage" the baby-making process.

In our culture, a satisfying sexual life can be used as a yardstick by which couples judge their relationship. When sex loses its passion, couples coping with infertility may feel that something has gone wrong with the relationship. In time, many come to accept this condition. Because they can no longer rely on love making as a way of achieving intimacy, they may realize that they have to find other ways of reinforcing and maintaining their union. Problems are more likely to persist when couples are unable to find alternatives for being close.

THE INFERTILE IDENTITY

As involvement in infertility treatment deepens, pinning down the exact nature of and appropriate treatments for infertility consumes increasing amounts of the couple's emotional and physical energy. The protracted focus on the infertility, with all of its psychological and social implications, typically causes individuals to begin to think about themselves differently: They may assume what has been called the *infertile identity* (Bassin, 1989; Greil, 1991; Hendricks, 1985). Although this becomes more pervasive in the Immersion phase, the process often begins in Mobilization, giving the clinician an opportunity to note it early and help clients develop ways to minimize its development.

> Alicia had her first miscarriage in the second trimester of pregnancy. The miscarriage occurred in the bathroom of an emergency room where the couple had rushed when heavy bleeding began. The hospital personnel's handling of the miscarriage was appalling. Alicia, for example, had to sit in a wheelchair for several hours holding the fetus in a cup on her lap, while other, "more important" emergencies took precedence. Thus, the couple's upsetting emergency room experience became the focus of that event.
>
> The couple's response to the first miscarriage was outrage and anger toward the medical system; they had no thoughts of infertility at that time. A second miscarriage led to infertility testing that showed no obvious problem with either partner. Alicia and Brad were relieved and still did not consider themselves infertile. However, after the third miscarriage, they decided they were infertile: "We realized that this was no longer normal." It was then that the infertile identity took hold and began to replace other self-perceptions. In fact, when the fetus of a fourth miscarriage was analyzed and found to have a genetic anomaly—"a fluke," the doctor said, one which "could happen to anyone,"—the infertile identity was too entrenched for Alicia and Brad to take his words to heart. The miscarriage was internalized as an event supporting the infertility.

In the process of taking on the infertile identity, couples move from perceiving infertility as a temporary obstruction that stands between the couple and parenthood to feeling like infertility is an enduring trait that resides within one or both partners. Infertility becomes "who I *am*" and "who we *are*," in that people come to feel that infertility constitutes the quintessential aspect of their identity. Because most people assume that the ability to reproduce comes naturally to everyone, the infertile identity also includes "who I am *not*" and "who we are *not*." People feel increasingly defective, deficient, deviant, and/or diseased, less masculine/feminine, and less adult. Often this profound sense of defect produces a host of negative thoughts. For example, many feel punished and/or ill-fated. In terms of their relationships to others, they feel like outsiders or aliens, not only within their families of origin but in our child-centered society.

> "Everything I see reminds me of kids," said Laura. "In the past I used to imagine how it was going to be me. . . . If I saw a pregnant woman, I'd think, 'I'm going to be like her, one day my body's going to have a big round belly like hers' . . . if I saw a woman with a carriage, I'd think I'd be doing that one day. . . . That's all gone now. But there's nothing else in its place. . . . I feel empty."

Infertility acts as a magnet, drawing negative self-perceptions to the fore. Many gender-based assumptions about reproduction come to be directly linked to the infertility; other negative self-perceptions are idiosyncratic. One woman was born with a congenital heart defect, which was later corrected with surgery. When she was diagnosed with infertility, she found herself overwhelmed with old feelings of abnormality, deformity, and disability.

Later, as the failures to get pregnant mount, any number of self-deprecating thoughts associated with failure and the loss of control may emerge. The inability to conceive in spite of seemingly heroic efforts on the part of the medical team can increase a person's sense that he or she is less competent, less successful, and perhaps even less worthy than others. At the same time, existing strengths, which had in the past contributed to a positive self-regard, no longer seem as meaningful as the ability to have a baby. Compared with the seemingly insurmountable obstacle of infertility, talents and skills may be disparaged:

> As one man said: "A part of my self image as a man who's creator and father is not there in terms of the physical aspect of it."

> "Yeah, it's just there all the time," said Danielle, "and I have to constantly be fighting and saying, 'All right, well, I'm not going to think of myself as an infertile woman right now, I'm going to be, you know, an architect drafting this plan.' But it requires that kind of constant focusing."

Gender Differences

Femininity and Masculinity

Our culture is permeated with messages in which femininity and masculinity are linked to fecundity; conversely, a host of negative gender connotations are connected to infertility and sterility. Thus, success at reproducing is typically felt to be a fundamental gauge of one's man- or womanhood. It is difficult, therefore, for those who struggle with infertility to avoid the idea that they are grievously flawed: "What are those people called? Androgynous I think—the kind that are neither male or female . . . that's how I see myself."

Significant differences exist between men and women depending on the gender of the partner who carries the infertility factor. Women tend to feel less feminine even when their partners are the ones who are diagnosed as infertile (Greil, 1991; Mathews & Mathews, 1993; Wirtberg, 1992). The woman with the congenital heart defect cited above took on the infertile identity in spite of the fact that it was actually her husband who was the carrier of the infertility factor; however, women need not have had histories of physical problems to react in this way. The following is a fairly typical reaction:

> "I know his sperm's the problem, but because I can't get pregnant and have a baby, I don't feel like a woman. . . . I know there's nothing physically wrong with me, but unless I have a baby, I won't feel like I fulfilled my destiny. . . . It sounds really crazy, but I sometimes feel like if I were more of a woman, I could make up for his problem."

Conversely, when women carry the infertility factor, their husbands' sense of manliness remains relatively intact (Abbey et al., 1992; Berg et al., 1991; Wirtberg, 1992): "I don't feel less manly, you know, less masculine. What I do feel is helpless, bad for her because I can't help with this problem." Men's apprehensions about their manliness are far more likely to arise when they carry the infertility factor, because power and potency are traditionally linked with a man's ability to sire offspring. Men, who prior to the diagnosis of infertility may have seen themselves as relatively "liberated" from gender stereotypes, are often chagrined to find that their male identity had been so closely linked with procreation; they may feel less manly when diagnosed as either being sterile or having a problem producing or delivering sperm: "I'm a total failure as a man. Getting a woman pregnant's pretty basic, isn't it? I thought that I wasn't affected by all that macho b.s., but I can't help it, I just don't feel like a man, a real man."

Motherhood and Fatherhood

The role of mother has traditionally been viewed as integral to the definition of what is female, whereas fatherhood has been less central to men's definition of themselves as male. Although recent changes in how members of our society view themselves have had some impact on these gender definitions, infertility often reveals how entrenched the traditional views are: "You know, I thought I was more 'liberated' . . . different from my own mother," Janet said. "But when I found I couldn't be a mother, I found out just how much I was primed to be one. . . . Compared to having a baby, all my other accomplishments seem trivial. . . . Being a mother is what it's all about."

In comparison, the following is an example of a man's self-perception vis-à-vis infertility and fatherhood: "It's bad, I'm very disappointed. . . . I feel devastated when I think about not having kids of my own, but I don't feel like there's something wrong with me or that I won't be a man if I can't be a father."

If individuals have reason to doubt their adequacy as potential parents, the diagnosis of infertility may serve to intensify the conviction that they are not suited to have children: "I always wondered whether I'd be a good father, my own father being the way he was [distant and critical]. He didn't know the first thing about being a father. . . . Now I feel like this could be nature's way of telling me to forget it, [that] I just won't make it as a father."

Body Identity

Women struggling with infertility are likely to have a host of negative feelings about their bodies and themselves, regardless of whether or not they are the infertile partner (Greil, 1991). They often feel that their bodies are defective or abnormal, that they are not womanly or feminine, and that they do not measure up to women who can produce children. These powerful feelings may spill over into an all-encompassing negative self-perception. Women may, for example, transport their feelings of inadequacy, incompleteness, and defect into their worklife and relationships: "At first we felt this was something we could lick. . . . I don't know how it happened, but more and more it seemed like it was me, not the infertility, that was the enemy. I could never feel it was 'just my body,' that somehow I was okay. . . . My body—that's a pretty big part of me. It is me!"

As mentioned earlier, men whose wives are the carriers of the infertility factor tend not to assume the infertile identity. But, because a noncarrier male is part of a couple that is not able to produce a baby, he may worry that others see him as less masculine. In one situation, a husband who was fertile worried that his family thought he was the carrier of the infertility. Because of his concern for how others perceived him, he broke his agreement with his wife not to reveal the carrier status and told his relatives that he "checked out fine," in order to correct his family's assumption. Not all men are so distressed. In a similar situation, for example, a noncarrier husband was annoyed that his family assumed he was the carrier, but he felt more amusement than injury and made no efforts to correct his relatives' assumption.

Age, Identity, and Infertility

Whereas men's fertility is relatively unaffected as they grow older, there is an inverse correlation between age and fertility for women. Accordingly, the infertile identity may have particularly strong meaning for older women (Harbour, 1997): "There's just no good time to find out you're infertile. . . . Before I got diagnosed, I thought, 'Sure I'm getting older,' but now I feel like I'm over the hill." First, they are older; second, they cannot have a baby: Thus, they may feel a dual impact from the losses associated with aging: "I feel just like my much older friends who are dealing with menopause. . . . It's nature's way of saying, 'Forget it as a woman.' " In contrast, younger women who learn they are infertile are less inclined to feel the impact of aging. However, they may take on other profound and pervasive aspects of the infertile identity, especially the sense of defect, deficiency, and deviance. In addition, whereas an older woman has had many years to enjoy her femininity and womanliness, a younger women diagnosed as infertile has had fewer years in which to define her womanhood," particularly regarding her sex life.

THE COUPLE AND THE SUPPORT SYSTEM

Distressed and overwhelmed by the necessity of medical involvement in getting pregnant, partners may turn toward family members, friends, associates, or, indeed, anyone who will listen. On the one hand, having a supportive person, or group of persons to lean on during the ordeal of infertility can be very helpful (Abbey et al., 1992; Greil, 1991). On the other hand, at this stage, many couples hope that the infertility will be relatively short-lived, and so they talk openly, often revealing many intimate details about their situation, and they may later regret the flood of information they shared during the early stages of infertility (Sandelowski & Jones, 1986). The identity of the carrier of the infertility factor (i.e., whether it is the wife or the husband) is information that some couples later wish they had not shared so freely. Furthermore, few couples imagine that they may eventually use donor gametes to have a baby. If this comes to pass, the couple may be concerned about how others' knowledge of this information will affect the perception and treatment of the child and themselves. Couples often regret not having restricted the information to a smaller set of family and friends.

> Anthony and Gabriella were Italian American, and Anthony's perception of his virility had been strongly affected by his diagnosis of male infertility. In order to shelter her husband from other people's reactions, Gabriella told her family and friends it was she who was infertile. At a family barbecue, her father approached Anthony and said he and his family would understand if Anthony wanted to divorce Gabriella because she could not produce any children.

In contrast to this open stance, some couples have deep misgivings about how the news of their infertility will be received by others. If these couples feel more private about their reproductive lives, or that there is something embarrassing or shameful about infertility, they may keep their distress to themselves. Here, too, there may be consequences further down the road. A pattern of isolation, which is initially restricted to the infertility, may increasingly come to govern their relationships with others as the infertility takes over their lives during the Immersion phase. As months, perhaps years, go by, the pattern can become fixed, with the couple becoming more and more isolated; many come to feel abandoned and misunderstood by family and friends, and, if part of their reticence to tell people about their condition is grounded in shame, the secrecy surrounding the infertility deepens the shame further. The couple's social network, unaware of what they are going through, are at a loss to understand how to relate to them. Friends and family may withdraw or try to find out what is going on; the withdrawal can exacerbate the couple's isolation, whereas inquiries about the couple's plans for having children can feel intrusive.

THE COUPLE AND THE MEDICAL SYSTEM

The Couple–Physician Relationship

According to one client in the Infertility Project, when couples seek infertility treatments, the "deal is that you hand your life over to the docs." Although dramatic, this description captures the essence of the contract between the couple and the physician: For the infertility treatments to be effective, it is necessary to subjugate significant areas of one's life to the exigencies of medical protocols (Berg & Wilson, 1991). Thus, in addition to the time, money, and energy required to undergo the testing and treatments for infertility, there are emotional sacrifices as well. The perception of lost control is a common experience among those undergoing infertility treatments (Bernstein, Mattonx, & Kellner, 1988).

Once couples enter the medical arena, they form a whole new set of relationships with doctors, nurses, lab technicians, and receptionists. The physician–patient relationship assumes great importance in the overall encounter with infertility (Burns, 1990; McDaniel et al., 1992). Many patients, impressed or intimidated by the doctors' authority and professional detachment, are inclined to give up their own autonomy in the face of the doctors' superior knowledge and expertise:

> "When we first met with the doctor, I felt like we were having an audience with the Pope. I don't mean that as a joke; I was filled with that kind of awe. . . . It was a solemn moment when he told us what he thought was wrong and what the odds of each procedure were."

When patients idolize their infertility specialist, they may have difficulty sorting out their preferences and/or questioning their doctor. Later, if treatments fail, they may feel disillusioned and even betrayed by their doctor (Kraft et al., 1980).

Other infertility patients may be more adversarial in their early encounters with their doctors. However, even patients who are more skeptical about the omnipotence of physicians in general and dubious about infertility specialists' profit motives in particular tend to avoid challenging their doctors. Couples may be afraid that if they ask too many questions (especially about how the doctor computes his or her success ratios or the costs of treatment) their physician will withhold treatments or be less aggressive in attacking the infertility due to concerns about the patients' emotional stability. Couples may try to be "good patients," suppressing or downplaying anything that might be construed as criticism of the physician. Unfortunately, this relational pattern with the physician may persist throughout the next phase, Immersion, when the physician–patient relationship becomes paramount. This frame of mind can have a negative impact on couples' ability to process the profound decisions they may confront later on.

The physician–patient relationship is characteristically asymmetrical in that the doctor exercises more control over the course and outcome of the treatment than does the patient. Furthermore, because most infertility specialists are men, and most infertility treatments pertain to women, the imbalance in this relationship tends to be reinforced by the gender archetypes of forceful men and passive women.

However, any notion that infertility patients are powerless is inaccurate. Most find strategies to exert some control over the relationship. They may educate themselves about every aspect of their treatment (many surf the Internet in search of current infertility protocols), question their physicians' choices, insist on modifications in protocols, and as Greil (1991) has noted, even misinform their physicians about how long they had tried to become pregnant. Furthermore, with the proliferation of and competition among infertility clinics, the threat of "taking our business elsewhere" may give couples the feeling that they have some leverage over their treatment.

When men accompany women to medical appointments, they may be seen by the physicians as minor players because they are not the primary patients, or they may be treated with greater deference than their partners simply because they are men. Either circumstance is likely to have ramifications for the couple.

Those who feel they must "present a good face" to their doctors tend to conceal their anxiety, sadness, disappointment, anger, and grief (Mahlstedt, 1985; Sandelowski & Jones, 1986), feelings that are generally more intense in the Immersion phase but may already be present in Mobilization. Couples who are struggling with infertility depend on the physician to help them achieve the goal of having a baby; this often becomes the couple's pragmatic reason to contain any hostility that arises.

However, because anger is often the trigger that motivates patients to question or disagree with a physician's recommendations or performance, infertility patients and their partners are at risk of being overly compliant regarding the course of treatment, the extent of treatment, and the number of times to try a procedure. Often, it is only during the Resolution phase, if no pregnancy has been achieved, that an emotional reckoning takes place. At that point, when couples have forfeited so much without having a child, intense feelings of disappointment and anger may surface: "We can't help feeling betrayed . . . we did everything the doctor said; he seemed so positive. . . . Is it wrong to feel he failed us?"

Triangulation

Triangulation (Bowen, 1976) in the physician–patient relationship occurs when the doctor and one member of the couple ally subtly against the other partner. For example, the woman may become very involved with the doctor, perhaps idolizing him or her. She may feel a bond with the doctor because of both the intimate nature of the medical procedures and also the special attention that she is receiving; in addition, she may feel as though the doctor is more responsive than her partner to her concerns about infertility. In this scenario, the man may feel as though he is excluded from the inner circle, that the doctor has in some way usurped his place as his wife's closest confidant, while he, the husband, is a mere "sperm donor." Alternatively, the doctor and the husband may be in collusion, particularly in the early phases, when both the doctor and husband may belittle the wife's concerns about infertility. One way to minimize problematic triangles is for both partners to attend as many doctor appointments together as possible. Another way is to encourage partners to discuss the difficult issues infertility raises.

In general, although these issues may not be as pronounced during Mobilization, it is useful to explore and address them early on so that as the couple enters the Immersion phase they will be better prepared to cope with the overwhelming nature of the medical involvement at that time. In addition, with their relationship as a couple strengthened, they will be able to function in supportive and nurturing roles, rather than being forced apart by the pressures of the more intensive medical procedures.

6

_⌒_

THERAPEUTIC APPROACH
IN THE MOBILIZATION PHASE

"I moved my office to my house so I could be home
with the baby and the pregnancy and the whole thing.
And suddenly I was left kinda with no prospect for a
baby, sitting there alone with my job in this big house."

Couples begin to experience significant distress during the Mobilization
phase, although it is not as intense as what usually occurs during Immersion. Because couples are not yet submerged in the most stressful and
time-consuming phase of medical treatment, therapists have a unique
opportunity during Mobilization to lay the groundwork for healthy patterns in the partner's relationships with the medical system, their family
and friends, and each other.

PRESENTING PROBLEM

Couples in the Mobilization phase are more likely to come for therapy
than couples in the Dawning phase. The disconcerting diagnosis of infertility, decreased sexual pleasure, and the prospect of never having a
genetically related baby place great stress on a relationship, and individual partners or couples may be troubled by the distressing feelings
aroused by the meaning of infertility. During Mobilization, marriages

start to show the strain, and some couples begin to question whether they should remain married at all. This concern seems especially compelling for couples whose marriages are primarily predicated on having children together.

RESPECT AND LIMIT THE IMPACT
OF THE INFERTILITY

Acknowledging Infertility's Power

Infertility is a serious crisis. If poorly handled, infertility can overshadow the couple's postinfertile life, affecting not only the couple but any children that subsequently become a part of the family. Given the various tangible and intangible stressors, couples are best able to make the appropriate accommodations to the infertility when they are aware of its effect on their lives and they acknowledge its power.

Although couples may understand that their distress is rooted in the infertility, and may be able to point to the acute stressors (e.g., failed pregnancies), on an emotional level in their day-to-day lives they begin to feel incompetent, defective, and punished. Without fully understanding the impact of infertility on their lives, as the partners' anguish increases, they often blame themselves or each other for the distress they are experiencing. Furthermore, once they are caught in the vortex of infertility, there is rarely time for couples to step back and recognize that infertility has distorted their perceptions of themselves, their partners, and life in general, thereby increasing their distress.

With an awareness of the influence infertility has over couples—the core issues that arise and the phases through which couples pass in their encounter with infertility—the therapist can help couples recognize and deal with their formidable adversary. He or she can serve as a guide, reminding couples to pay attention to and respect the many ways infertility impacts on their lives: "More important than any of the particular feelings discussed in therapy was the act of going together. It fostered a closeness that was largely absent in our daily life. . . . I am sure that the therapy helped bridge the gap I felt between us at home."

It is important to normalize the clients' many uncomfortable feelings by suggesting that these are common responses to the crisis of infertility. Partners may describe feeling out of control or defective, reveal doubts about their ability to parent, or disclose that they feel unfeminine or unmasculine. At this juncture, the clinician can share the similar experiences of other couples who have faced infertility. By thus universalizing the reactions to the current crisis, the therapist provides a community for the couple.

Externalize the Infertility

If infertility is the first major crisis in the partners' life together, they may soon discover their relationship's weakest and strongest elements. When undiscovered or underutilized assets seem overshadowed by problematic interpersonal dynamics, the clinician can play a role in helping the partners locate and utilize their strengths while highlighting the particular stressors that are a part of coping with infertility.

In particular, the clinician can help couples to externalize the infertility (White, 1989) and thereby separate the infertility from their identity. Thus, as discussed in Chapter 2, if they are thinking or saying, "I am/ he or she is/ we are infertile," the clinician can encourage them to shift this perception to "We are struggling with infertility; we are experiencing infertility." When provided with this perspective, couples are more able to hold onto the idea basic to all our treatment: that *infertility*, not the *relationship*, is the problem. Even though the physical symptom resides within one partner, conceptualizing it as an external adversary helps the couple join together and regain the partnership that may have been lost: "When I thought of myself as defective, I just wanted to pull away. But when I saw infertility as our mutual enemy, we pulled together."

THE THERAPIST'S ROLE

As stated before but worth reemphasizing, the clinician must be aware of his or her own biases regarding children and parenting and the value of genetic connections. If, for example, the clinician does not value parenting and children very highly, he or she may be less sympathetic about the couple's distress and may have trouble understanding why the couple is willing to undergo the ordeal of infertility procedures. If, on the other hand, the clinician believes that having a child is of paramount importance, he or she may encourage the couple to move quickly to a solution for the infertility. He or she would tend to talk about what the next procedure is and when they are planning to do it, rather than asking the clients what the value of children is for them, how much they want children, and what they are willing to pay, both emotionally and financially. The therapist thus avoids confronting uncomfortable feelings (e.g., his or her own fear of childlessness, the couple's grief, etc.), dealing with the couple's losses, and exploring what the couple really wants.

A related pitfall is that the therapist may follow the lead of the most enthusiastic member, neglecting to determine whether or not the other partner is comfortable with proceeding. One partner may be very vocal and enthusiastic while the silent partner may be concealing a great deal of pain. In general, the therapist needs to check that the partners are in agreement. Each partner may approach the complex issues of infertility according to a different schedule. When one partner needs more time, the clinician must be aware of the tendency to see that client as resistant. It is important not to criticize the hesitant partner or to assume, for example, that he or she is being obstructive. Hesitation and the need to think things over before taking action are normal reactions to the process of infertility treatment and should not automatically be interpreted as an indication that that partner does not want a child. Regarding couples' relationships with doctors, the therapist may hesitate to encourage couples to be informed consumers of infertility treatments for two reasons. First, he or she may not know the details of the treatments available. To best serve clients, it is essential to be conversant with this subject, and we have provided a brief medical overview in the Appendix. Second, therapists themselves may be overly compliant in the medical arena; one of us learned from participating in the Infertility Project to be more assertive with her own doctors. Thus, the therapist must be aware of his or her own attitudes about the sanctity of the medical profession and the doctor's role. The therapist must also question personal beliefs about infertility treatments, that is, whether he or she considers them natural extensions or artificial manipulations of the reproductive process. Clinicians must be vigilant in questioning their own assumptions about what is "right" or "natural" with regard to medical procedures, parenting, and children.

LOCATE THE COUPLE ON THE TRAJECTORY

Eliciting the Story

Eliciting the couple's infertility story pays tribute to and validates the couple's struggle; thus, telling the story is a healing ritual in and of itself. It is important to begin with an open-ended invitation, such as "Tell me your story," or "What have you been through?" As with asking about someone's surgery or experience of childbirth, people are usually eager to recount their experience with infertility. Couples may begin tentatively, but as they recognize that the clinician is familiar with the medical information they begin to speak more freely. They are usually relieved that they do not have to explain all the technical information, and they develop confidence that the therapist will understand them. Also, by being familiar with the medical procedures, he or she will be aware that certain procedures, such as a hysterosalpingogram, are painful and invasive, and will understand the client's level of affect. However, it is important for the therapist not to let his or her assumptions get in the way of asking about the client's own experiences with these medical procedures.

As in all couple therapy, it is vital to hear each partner's story, as well as each one's perception of the problem and any feelings attached to it. It is necessary to look for differences in the story as well as potential conflicts. In hearing the story, the clinician can begin to get an idea of when the stresses began to build, whether there was a particular procedure that precipitated the crisis, and what is unique in this couple's reaction to the infertility experience. He or she also begins to get an idea of the partners' emotional states and the couple dynamics. For example, are they together in the process? Is only one partner worrying? Is only one of them grieving about the miscarriages? Was one partner ahead from the start, and is the other playing catch-up? This process helps the clinician to join with the couple and understand their particular ordeal.

Evoking the Future

Couples in Mobilization tend to be action oriented and optimistic. In addition, they may already be caught up in the "treadmill of treatment" that is a hallmark of Immersion, when couples often move unthinkingly from one test or treatment to the next. It is helpful for couples to take some time to consider the implications of their actions, and to ask themselves how far they are willing to go in pursuing pregnancy. Asking these questions relatively early on may help prevent couples from rushing ahead into expensive and psychologically complex treatments and making poor choices. Questions regarding the meaning and value of children and parenting are important to review at this time (see Chapters 2 & 4). In addition, the therapist can address the following areas: (1) levels of intervention, and (2) expenditures of time, money, and effort. Opening up these discussions enables couples to set some preliminary limits and to have a road map before they enter the daunting territory of Immersion.

Regarding levels of intervention, the clinician can ask some of the following questions:

- What level of invasiveness are you willing to tolerate, and do you (partner) agree?
- Which one of you would be more likely to use donor gametes? What reservations do each of you have, and how do you deal with these differences?

Questions regarding expenditures of time, money, and effort are as follows:

- Which of you feels more strongly about having children? How long are you willing to keep trying?

- Who is more worried about putting your savings at risk?
- If you find infertility and its treatments very distressing, how much do you think you can tolerate?
- Which of you would be the first to think about ending medical treatment?

WORKING WITH THE COUPLE: THERAPEUTIC ISSUES, TECHNIQUES, AND STRATEGIES

As couples begin their involvement with the medical system, infertility comes to occupy an increasingly prominent place in their lives until, by the time they are in the Immersion phase, it may become their sole focus. Therefore, as clinicians, we have a unique opportunity during the Mobilization phase to preserve the non-infertility-related activities in couples' lives. Although this intervention may become imperative in Immersion, during Mobilization it can serve as a preventative, helping the couple to maintain a balance in the social, personal, and sexual arenas of their lives.

Time In/Time Out

As discussed in Chapter 2, a useful concept in working with infertility, drawn from the work in chronic illness, is to *make a place for infertility and keep infertility in its place* (Gonzalez, Steinglass, & Reiss, 1989). A specific technique for managing the emotional upheavals is the use of *time in/time out* from the infertility (Bombardieri, 1983). The couple can take time to concentrate on the infertility, but alternate this with much-needed respites. This technique can be applied specifically to the sexual relationship and also to other couple activities, and can be initiated in any phase of infertility, as needed. However, this may be problematic when a woman is older and feels she does not want to use valuable time, or if it goes against either of the couple's coping styles. In addition, partners may not feel like having fun together until they voice some of their worry or conflict.

Sex

The clinician can inquire about the couple's sex life both before infertility and currently. If, as so often happens, problems have arisen in relation to the timing of intercourse with the woman's ovulation cycle, the clinician can introduce the idea of sex for pleasure and intimacy versus sex for reproduction. By setting aside the baby-making agenda and enjoying sex for its own sake, the couple can often revive their pleasure in each other as sexual partners.

EXPLORE COUPLES' BELIEF SYSTEMS

The prospect of infertility is likely to trigger each partner's core beliefs, basic assumptions, and world views. While the physician searches for a physical explanation for the infertility, people tend to come to their own conclusions, which may have little to do with biology and much to do with their own idiosyncratic beliefs. These beliefs may include the meaning and value they attach to children and parenthood (see Chapters 2 & 4), as well as what being unable to have children and to experience parenthood means to them. Themes of defectiveness, inferiority, guilt, and retribution often emerge.

The clinician can engage the couple in discussing ways of curtailing shame by reframing the meaning of infertility. This early intervention on the part of the clinician limits the negative impact of infertility on each partner and the couple. In order to explore these important themes, the clinician can ask the couple for their thoughts on a wide range of infertility-related subjects (see also Chapter 2):

- What different beliefs do you have regarding the carrier versus the noncarrier of infertility?
- Which one of you feels more affected in your sense of being a woman or a man?
- Who holds the stronger belief that one cannot be an adult without being a parent?
- Which one of you feels most deprived when among family and friends?

It is important with regard to the expectation of parenthood to remember that one's identity includes the expected future self. When this future self is blocked, as in infertility or chronic illness (Sandelowski, 1993), this affects the view of the current self. Once these destructive beliefs have been brought to light, the clinician can help to minimize angry, painful, shameful legacies by addressing and reframing them (see also Chapter 2).

- Would you see yourself differently if you saw infertility as bad luck instead of a sign you are defective?
- How would that different view affect the way you function in your marriage and in the world?

FACILITATE MOURNING

Recognizing Losses

The therapist can assume that couples are experiencing loss of control over their bodies and reproductive life. As couples tell their stories, he or she helps them identify their losses and validates their feelings. If couples are unaware of any losses, the therapist can make a universal statement such as "Many couples feel very out of control during infertility treatment. Is that something you feel?" In this way, he or she articulates clients' unspoken, perhaps unrecognized distress.

Infertility losses will often be expressed as anger. One can assume that couples may feel a great deal of sadness at the loss of what they hoped would be a "normal" conception and of control over their reproductive life, and that the anger is a way to avoid the experience of loss. For some, the physician may be the primary target; for others, it may be friends, family, or the partner. To help identify the impact of the losses on the relationship, the clinician can ask questions such as the following:

- What impact does your sadness have on the relationship?
- If you let yourself get sad right now, which of you would have a harder time?

It may be important to find out what other life experiences might be related to their reactions to the infertility and to discover how they have handled these crises in the past. This becomes an opportunity to draw upon previous strengths and develop new coping strategies.

EXPLORE THE RELATIONSHIP WITH THE SUPPORT SYSTEM

As family systems clinicians, we are likely to assume that people can better cope with life crises such as infertility when they have the support of their social networks. However, although those who struggle with infertility benefit from the support of friends and family, clinicians can play an important role in helping couples make prudent decisions about what kinds of information to share with whom (see Chapter 5).

When couples are unsure about what or how much to tell others, we have found it useful to introduce the distinction that Karpel (1980) makes between matters that are "private" and those that are "secret." Particularly meaningful to this distinction is the concept of the "relevance of the information for the unaware" (p. 298). For example, the relevance of information is important when considering whether to disclose adoption or donor conception to a child, for keeping either secret might be damaging to the child (see Chapters 12 and 14 for in-depth discussion of disclosure). However, whether to discuss infertility problems with family members, friends, or acquaintances is an issue of privacy, in that there are many people for whom the details of a couple's infertility experience are not relevant.

Some couples prefer to keep the information regarding which partner carries the infertility factor private from the start; others make that information public. For the latter group, if it turns out that they never become pregnant, they may wish that the carrier's status was not general knowledge.

Conversely, when couples choose to share very few facts about their infertility with their families and friends, it is useful for the clinician to determine whether they are usually reticent about discussing personal matters or if shame has begun to affect their self-perceptions.

When partners disagree about whether to let others know about their medical status and treatments, or about whom and what to tell, the clinician can help them locate any underlying beliefs and feelings of shame that may be creating tensions. When these beliefs are out in the open, the partners are more able to discuss their disagreements and make decisions that respect each partner's way of thinking.

In thinking about couples' relationships with their families and friends, it is important for the clinician to help couples take a step back from the present crisis and ask what life might be like if the infertility continues for longer than they expect:

- If the infertility were to last for many months or longer, who are the people that you would like to have in your support network?
- Who should be privy to information regarding your diagnosis and treatments?
- Who might best be left out of the information loop?
- Bearing in mind that once information is disclosed, it cannot always be restricted, how much and what kind of information is appropriate to share?

Another useful technique for couples to consider is telling their friends and family that "just for now" they will not be available to attend family celebrations and get-togethers that are potentially painful. In this way, couples can protect themselves from having to present a happy demeanor when in fact they are full of grief and jealousy for what others have and they do not, such as at child-centered family celebrations. At the same time, they can preserve their relationships with those close to them, assuring their friends and family that this need to separate is only temporary. The couple's temporary or selective withdrawal can be conceptualized as a choice for privacy about a painful subject (Schaffer & Diamond, 1993); however, the therapist must also discuss obtaining appropriate support from more understanding friends and family members, and from RESOLVE.

EXPLORE THE RELATIONSHIP
WITH THE MEDICAL SYSTEM

The physician–patient relationship, set in motion at the start of the infertility consultation, is likely to become the prevailing pattern in later phases. It is helpful to address this early in infertility as patients may feel too vulnerable later on to rectify any communication problems and clashes that develop with their infertility specialists.

Although patients may not bring up the issue themselves, by empowering them to ask questions of their doctors, the therapist enables them to be more informed consumers of infertility services. The clinician can inquire about the physician–patient relationship using some of the following questions, and explain why establishing a workable dynamic early on may be an important part of coping with the infertility.

> Are you comfortable with your doctor?
> Are you able to speak freely to him or her?
> Are your concerns about infertility understood and taken seriously?
> Are you treated with respect?
> Are you comfortable asking your physician for information?
> Do you feel you can question your doctor's recommendations?

A Couples Approach to the Medical System

As mentioned earlier, the clinician can suggest that the partners visit the physician together (Berger et al., 1995). By taking a conjoint approach to matters of reproduction at this early juncture, the couple is in a better position to handle problems further down the road. The clinician may want to say that when a man accompanies his partner to the doctor's office he is not only lending support, but is also hearing all information first-hand and may have his questions answered directly; confusion and disagreement between partners, therefore, is less likely to develop. The husband's attendance is especially important for the woman, as her body is often the site of the medical procedures. His presence helps to mitigate the feelings that she is shouldering the burden alone.

END OF MOBILIZATION

"We were already up to our ankles in all the tests; we decided to wade in a little further."

The transition between the investigation of medical treatment options and the decision to enter the medical arena for treatment is often blurred. In part this is due to the nature of the medical assessments. A laparoscopy, for example, is both a diagnostic and remedial intervention. When physicians meet with the couple to discuss the findings, they pair the diagnoses with appropriate treatment options. Therefore, when the couple receives the diagnosis, they may be told what they can do about it. If, for example, the man's sperm count is found to be low, donor insemination (DI) or intracytoplasmic sperm injection (ICSI; see the Appendix for descriptions of medical procedures) may be suggested. Similarly, if the woman's tubes are damaged, *in vitro* fertilization (IVF) is often the proposed treatment.

Knowing that the biological clock is ticking, some couples feel pressure to leap into medical treatments without taking time to step back and weigh each choice and its possible consequences. Others carefully consider the next steps before entering the medical arena. Few fully realize what lies ahead. Grief and sadness are deferred; so long as medicine holds out the promise of a pregnancy, couples can ignore the possibility that they may not become pregnant and have a genetically related child.

7

⬿

COUPLE ISSUES IN THE EARLY AND MIDDLE IMMERSION PHASE

> "It's like walking into a forest. . . . Once you're in it, you keep walking because you believe that each step will bring you closer to the other side. It takes a while before you realize you might be going around in circles and [begin to] worry if you'll ever get out."

CHARACTERISTICS OF IMMERSION

In the Immersion phase, couples become increasingly absorbed in the world of medical treatment. Relatively simple, inexpensive procedures give way to more complicated, costly treatments. A couple's decision to proceed may be propelled not only by the wish to have a child, but also by the desire to avoid the pain of loss that is implicit in the termination of treatment. Consequently, some couples may undertake more invasive and financially burdensome procedures than they would otherwise. The social isolation seen in Mobilization becomes more pronounced, and the infertile identity takes a firm hold, driving out other interests and activities in the couple's life. The alternating cycle of hope (with each new protocol) and despair (with each treatment failure) creates tremendous distress, and the couple relationship is subjected to acute pressures.

In late Immersion, hope may increasingly give way to despair; in addition, couples may confront a major treatment decision: whether or not to use donor gametes. This complex subphase will be discussed in Chapters 9 and 10. But, at the start of Immersion, few realize how long their journey may last or how much distress they may encounter: "We seemed to have just slipped into it. We were just having some tests to see if there was a problem. . . . It seems like the next thing we knew, we were fully into it and going for broke."

MEDICAL PROCEDURES

Infertility specialists are now able to find physiological explanations for most infertility. However, many couples have to wait months or years before a diagnosis is found, and 10-15% never learn the reason for their inability to conceive.

A couple may be presented with many options during the Immersion phase. Before suggesting assisted reproductive technology (ART) such as IVF, the doctor will often pursue less invasive and less expensive procedures, including intrauterine insemination (IUI) and hormonal therapy (Berger et al., 1995; see also the Appendix for a detailed description of medical procedures). Exploratory surgery such as laparoscopy and hysteroscopy may reveal problems that can be treated during the procedure. Male factor infertility may be treated with IUI, surgery to correct varicoceles or other structural abnormalities, and, in rare cases, hormonal therapy (Marrs, 1997).

If these treatments have been ineffective, the physician may propose ART, and the couple may undergo IVF, gamete intrafallopian transfer (GIFT), zygote intrafallopian transfer (ZIFT), and/or ICSI. Following these procedures, the doctors will probably cryopreserve (freeze) any unused embryos for possible later use by the couple.

Even after a diagnosis is made, there is no guarantee that any protocol will succeed. Although highly specialized treatments are now available for many previously irremediable conditions, no matter how advanced the procedure, physicians still face a singularly complex and unpredictable organism—the human body. Protocols with the best track records may fail, whereas those with low success rates may be effective after only one or two tries. In general, success rates remain disappointing (see Table 1, Appendix).

THE CRISIS AND TRAUMA OF INFERTILITY

The Limbo of Immersion

In most cultures, reproduction allows for the continuation of its people; in families, children carry on the family line. Childbearing, therefore is an essential, often definitive phase in a couple's life cycle. Unless partners have mutually decided to lead lives without children, or they plan to adopt, giving birth to genetically related offspring entitles them to become legitimate adult members of their society. For couples struggling with infertility, while others around them may be moving forward, they feel that they cannot do so until they have a baby. Couples are in a state of "active waiting," with much activity but little or no forward movement. Thus, many describe the Immersion phase as a time spent in limbo, an anxious waiting period marked by spurts of action, disappointing failures, and endless delays.

> Paul said he felt as though he were socked in by fog in an airport when he badly needed to get on his plane. "It doesn't feel like it's just an important business trip," he said. "It feels like my life depends on getting out of this place."

This state of limbo—being unable either to proceed or to go back to life before infertility—is compounded by the immersion in medical treatments. Preoccupied with these procedures, "we do not allow ourselves to realize how much we are forfeiting in order to get pregnant," as Cheryl put it. Often, it is only with hindsight that couples realize the extent to which they became "sucked in," "completely taken over," "obsessed," and "consumed" by the infertility: "It was like quicksand, only we didn't know we were in it."

When infertility specialists can find no clear-cut diagnosis, the couple's sense of being stuck is that much more overwhelming. In these cases, physicians may prescribe treatments or perform medical interventions to enhance the couple's fertility, but without having pinpointed the cause, neither the doctors nor their patients can be sure that a particular protocol makes sense.

> "It feels like we're shooting in the dark," said Howard, "firing into an enemy . . . that might not even be where we think it is. . . . I worry what all this medication is doing to my wife; the costs are pretty astounding too. But how can we stop? Nobody's told us to forget it: 'Here's the problem. You're not going to get pregnant.' . . . I guess we'll keep firing till we run out of ammunition."

The Roller Coaster of Hope and Despair

Nearly every couple who struggles with infertility describes the extreme fluctuations of emotion that they undergo. The promise of a new treatment technique or a consultation with a different physician mitigates their hopelessness about having a baby, and even though a treatment trial has failed, the next one might succeed. The oscillations between hope and despair are so constant that many couples use the metaphor of a roller coaster to describe the radical shifts in their emotional state. One day their hopes soar, another day they are overcome with despair: "Neither of us ever can be sure how we're going to feel the next minute. . . . Sometimes my mood changes suddenly without warning, with or without the hormones; and sometimes it's the direct result of finding out bad news."

After experiencing several ups and downs on the roller coaster, couples often try to keep painful disappointments in check by lowering their expectations: "We're trying to keep our hopes real small, just in case it doesn't work. We don't want to set ourselves up for another crash like last time." However, every baby they see is a reminder of their desired goal, and each new procedure raises the hope that this may be the one that finally achieves that goal.

LOSS

During Immersion, prior losses are compounded by additional ones. Primary among them is the possible loss of creating a child together. As couples come to realize that this could be the outcome of their encounter with infertility, their sadness may be profound. Even though their worst fear—childlessness—has not yet happened, their distress in anticipation of the loss may be great (Sandelowski, 1993). This is often coupled with a unique kind of loss that Boss (1991) terms *ambiguous loss*, which has been noted in families with a member who is missing in action.[1] Although the member is physically absent, without evidence confirming the death, the member remains psychologically present. The uncertainty creates emotional ambiguity. With infertility, although the lost object (the child) never existed, the fantasized child assumes an emotional reality for the couples.

Control of Time

"It can get quite time consuming. Like right now, Evie's supposed to be taking . . . whatever it is . . . progesterone suppositories, twice a day for a half hour—so she is immobilized an hour a day.

---

[1]While visiting the Infertility Project, Boss noted that the couples with whom we worked were experiencing ambiguous loss.

So there she is, sitting there, feeling unpregnantly ... stuck.
There's the shots, the schlepping around ... and then, emotionally, I don't know, I mean it's always sort of there."

Infertility testing and treatments can interfere significantly with
couples' control over their time. For example, the man must go to the
doctor's office to provide sperm for testing and/or various procedures,
sometimes several times in a week. He may also wish to be present at
any insemination or ART transfer procedures and thus must ask for
additional time off from work.

Ed, an attorney, was scheduled to try an important case in court on
the day that Rhonna was scheduled for her embryo transfer. The
physician assured him that he would not need to be present, and
Rhonna said that she had been through enough procedures to feel
this was "no big deal." Ed, however, requested and was granted a
postponement by the judge. "If this is the one that takes," he said,
"I want to know that I was there at the beginning."

However, for the woman the demands are generally much more
intense. Initial ovulation testing is fairly undemanding and can be done
at home, but testing and treatment become progressively more time consuming. For example, most ART procedures require a cycle of injections
beginning on the first or second day after the onset of menstruation.
These must be done at the same time each day and are difficult to self-
administer; if the partner is reluctant to perform the injection, the
woman must either do it herself or enlist the help of a friend or neigh-
bor. Starting on the eighth day, the woman must have a sonogram every
morning until ovulation is imminent. At that time, she receives an injection of human menopausal gonadotropin (hMG; see the Appendix for a
description) and must return to the doctor's office 36 hours later to have
her eggs retrieved. This is usually an all-day procedure because either
general anesthesia or twilight sleep is necessary. If the eggs have been
fertilized, the woman must return to the doctor's office in 2 days for the
embryo transfer. Following the transfer, she must lie still in the office for
5–6 hours to allow for implantation. After 12 days, she must return for
a blood test to learn if the embryo(s) have implanted. Yet the statistical
rate of having a live birth from IVF is low, and there is a good chance all
the trouble may be for nothing.

The time spent away from work receiving infertility treatments can
leave little or no remaining time for maternity leave in the event of a successful pregnancy. Although many clinics open early in the morning to
accommodate work schedules, they are often located in major medical

centers, which are not likely to be close to clients' homes. If there is no infertility clinic nearby, women may travel to New York, California, Norfolk, VA (site of one of the earliest infertility clinics), or other distant locations for treatment. Women may be required to spend 2 weeks in the vicinity of the clinic, whereas men need only join them to provide sperm.

Loss of Innocence

Couples who face infertility often experience a loss of innocence—their sense that the world is a safe and just place and that life is basically good. During Immersion, these feelings are usually most pronounced.

> "A few months ago, we realized we reached a point of no return. Even if we have a baby, we've passed the place where we can just get back to our lives as they were before," said Brad. Alicia added, "Life has taken on a sadness and seriousness that I know will last even if we succeed at having a baby. . . . I feel like we lost our innocence."

Early Treatment Failure

Even when couples have been briefed by their physician about what to expect, the first few treatment failures are painful events because couples have not yet developed the ability to protect themselves from the pain of further losses: "I guess you have to really experience this kind of news; you can't really prepare yourself for it . . . but once you've felt that stab in the heart, you try to protect yourself better the next time." This is a time when hopes are up and defenses are down. Later treatment failures are also painful because, while hopes are down, defenses are never high enough to avoid facing the increasing probability of failure. The pain of treatment failures may discourage some couples from continuing the process. However, most will endure many more failures before their threshold is reached. Research (Boivan, Takefman, Tulandi, & Brender, 1995) indicates that it is the accumulation of these failures that contributes to the decision to abandon treatment.

Miscarriage

The miscarriage rate for all pregnancies is 20–25% (Marrs, 1997). If women who are not involved in infertility procedures miscarry during the first weeks of their pregnancies, they are rarely able to distinguish the event from their monthly menstruation. However, with IVF and related interventions, all of the early phases of fertilization, implantation, and gestation are monitored closely. Couples, therefore, immediately learn whether fertilization has occurred, how many eggs were fertilized, and whether implantation was successful.

Couples who have struggled with infertility may not only have especially strong feelings and fantasies regarding the developing life, but if a miscarriage or stillbirth occurs, because they know how difficult it will be to get pregnant again, their grief is amplified. Unfortunately, our culture offers no mourning rituals for couples grappling with repeated miscarriages, which has been termed the "forgotten grief" (Kirkley-Best & Kellner, 1982). After a miscarriage, the grief can be overwhelming. Many who thought they were keeping their feelings in check are often surprised at how deeply they experience their loss. Some hospitals compound the grief by placing a woman who has miscarried on a maternity ward, which is especially agonizing for infertility patients.

> "I was put in a room with another woman who miscarried too. She already had a child; she was upset but kept saying, 'I'm going to get pregnant right away, and I hope to be back here in a year to have my baby.' I couldn't comfort myself that way. . . . When I could go home, I walked down the hall and saw the nursery. I didn't feel like 'Next time it's my turn'; I felt that from now on, I'd probably be staring through the glass at other people's babies. Giving me a taste of pregnancy was a terrible trick nature played. I wonder if I'd be better off if it never happened."

Fortunately, other hospitals are changing these policies and even offer bereavement counseling for couples who have miscarried (McDaniel et al., 1992).

Anger, Blame, and Shame

In addition to grief, emotional responses to loss may include anger, frustration, and indignation. Individuals may be angry about their seemingly unjust fate and frustrated by the vagaries of human biology. Anger may be especially keen when doctors are unable to find a medical explanation for the infertility. Anger, shame, and blame are likely to overflow into the couple's relationship. At times, fertile partners have difficulty avoiding overt or covert references to the carrier's responsibility for the infertility:

> "It slips out sometimes, when I'm mad at him for something else, or after we've had another failure," said Deborah. Her husband, Sid, described it this way: "I think I walk around feeling guilty and hang-dog most of the time these days. I feel like I've done this ter-

rible thing to her, so even when we could be having an okay time, I'm especially sensitive to her gibes. . . . I either take it and get more depressed, or I snap back. . . . Sometimes I pick at little faults of hers. . . . I guess I'm trying not to feel like the only one with a problem."

Families, friends, acquaintances, or colleagues may also become targets for the couple's anger:

"I can't help it. I walk around mad at the world and mad at anyone who doesn't understand what we're going through. . . . How many times do I need to tell them? Still they'll say something like my cousin did the other night . . . she thought it was funny to say she'd gladly give me her kids for the weekend . . . so I'd see it wasn't all roses having children."

However, although anger can be an emotional refuge that temporarily keeps couples from falling into despair, it is usually not sustained in the face of the recurring sadness.

IMPACT ON THE COUPLE RELATIONSHIP

Secrecy and Protection

By introducing a climate of secrecy and withholding, the dynamic of *protection*—when partners conceal negative emotions and thoughts in an effort to protect each other—frequently puts a severe strain on the couple's ability to communicate. Because couples tend to be optimistic and action oriented in early Immersion, there is also a tendency to set disturbing feelings aside so that medical testing and treatment can progress.

An imbalance in medical involvement is typical of the Immersion phase: The man, unlike the woman, is spared most of the procedures. Therefore, he is subjected to less physical discomfort and pain, he is not subject to hormone-induced mood swings, and fewer limitations are placed on his travels and career. These differences are likely to produce difficulties within the couple's relationship. At the least, the imbalance may lead to resentment on the part of the woman because her partner is spared so much of the ordeal. Her partner, on the other hand, may feel guilty for being spared. When these feelings remain unexpressed, tensions and rifts may develop.

Partners also may have difficulty talking together about their losses. Sorting out one's own feelings can be difficult enough without having to express them to a partner who is already suffering. When couples stifle these powerful thoughts and feelings, they tend to withdraw from each other. The protection dynamic may then backfire as censored thoughts tend to magnify when unexpressed.

Protection often emerges in relation to who carries the infertility factor. As 85–90% of all infertility workups establish which partner is the carrier, once the couple is given the test results, each partner is likely to experience a variety of troubling feelings. The carrier often feels guilty and perhaps ashamed, whereas the noncarrier may be disappointed and angry with his or her partner. For example, when the man is the carrier, the woman may feel resentful, even bitter, about having to undergo life-disrupting and painful procedures that would not be necessary if he were fertile. The man, on the other hand, may feel guilty for being the source of her distress. A woman whose partner carries the infertility factor may be reluctant, even fiercely opposed, to express her grief in his presence. If the woman carries the infertility factor, she may feel responsible for the couple's problem and therefore not entitled to express her distress about the medical procedures.

Another dynamic at play vis-à-vis the carrier and noncarrier is that the carrier often feels less physically attractive and less masculine or feminine. It is especially difficult to deal with this diminished sense of one-self as a sexual being when carriers sense that their partners' sexual attraction has lessened.

> "I'm ashamed to say, but I find myself looking at him differently," said Elaine, who was carrying an ICSI pregnancy. "I see traits which seem feminine. . . . I think I always saw them, but now they disturb me."

> "I feel really terrible about this," said Tom. "I love her, but the fact that she can't get pregnant makes me find her less sexy."

When the reason for the infertility is interactive, one partner, typically the woman, may feel more at fault, or partners may blame each other in an effort to avoid taking on the infertile identity.

During Immersion, many people try to erect protective emotional barriers in order to shield themselves from embarrassment, loss of privacy, physical distress, repeated disappointments, and the insensitive remarks of others. However, these barriers may also prevent individuals from feeling their sense of loss.

After 2 years of fertility treatments, Renee thought of herself as an infertility veteran. "I can shop for a baby gift without feeling like I'm going to dissolve," she said. "I can't say I've accepted it though. I'm just numb I think. . . . I move through a lot of my life like a zombie; nothing seems to get to me any more."

But the protective walls are rarely impassable. An event or a random thought may penetrate the barrier and cause acute pain.

> Renee went to a matinee movie. At one point, a small child making her way to the end of the aisle passed in front of Renee, and Renee felt the child's hair touch her face. "I guests I didn't have time to get the walls up . . . and I started to sob. . . . I had to leave the theater."

Out of Synch

The length of time needed to grieve the losses of infertility varies from person to person. For this reason, partners may be emotionally out of synch. For example, one partner may cope best by getting busy and continuing treatment, whereas the other needs time to grieve. If a protocol is imminent, for example, the man may need time to grieve, but the woman knows that every day her eggs are getting a little older and her probability of infertility a little higher, so she feels the pressure and does not want to wait.

> Lorraine said, "While I know it makes emotional sense to give Howard time to recover from the miscarriage, we can't afford to lose the time." Howard responded, "The more she pressures me to get with the program, the harder it gets to deal with how I feel."

Each additional medical procedure may cause them to question their level of commitment to having children. They can be out of synch about this at the outset—for example, the woman wants children, and the man is less enthusiastic about having them—and the gap may widen with each repetition of a protocol. Alternatively, their positions may reverse, for example, the same man may get very excited about having a child just at the moment that the woman decides the treatment is too hard on her body and that she has had enough.

Couples may also have different ideas about how much money to spend on getting pregnant. One partner may feel that no expense is too great, whereas the other may be concerned about setting aside savings, for example, for the child's college education. Disagreements about this issue can be quite intense, sometimes triggering longstanding conflicts about money.

Gender Differences

Although the majority of couples with whom we work are dual-income families, like other researchers (Abbey et al., 1992; Berg et al., 1991; Wirtberg, 1992), we find that men tend to define themselves by their work and women by both their work and their expectations to become a mother one day or, with secondary infertility, to have another child or a particular family size.

At the workplace, women are more likely than men to be exposed to reminders that they are without children. They are invited to baby showers and tend to be aware of the other women who are taking maternity leave and having babies: "I used to find that work was my salvation; it was where I could throw myself into work and forget about the infertility for a while. But now I find I can't escape it. . . . Reminders are everywhere."

In contrast, even when men are reminded of a child-centered life, they seem to be less affected and can often avoid discussions about children without seeming evasive. Indeed, men often escape into their work: "It's a place in which to forget about all the trouble. . . . I find myself staying to finish a project as a way to avoid coming home and back to the misery." Ultimately, when infertility persists, and one's peers in the workplace are having children, it is the woman who shows, by her inability to become pregnant, that she is different from her coworkers—"They keep kidding me about how I better get started soon. They think I'm choosing this . . . that I'm not having a baby because I'm too selfish"—while the difference can go undetected for men.

In addition, when women have demanding, high-profile careers, infertility treatment can pose a substantial problem.

> Rita, an investment banker, traveled all over the country. Her IVF procedure required her to be at the doctor's office to measure blood levels, but during the same time period, she had business meetings scheduled out of town. She was thus faced with the choice of skipping the treatment or putting her career at risk.

Although men's work may suffer as the result of the stresses related to infertility, women's careers are placed in much greater jeopardy.

Sexual Relationship

During the Immersion phase, obstacles to a satisfying sex life intensify: the need to coordinate sex with ovulation, the association of sex with unsuccessful attempts to get pregnant, performance anxiety, loss of desire, and the diminution of the sense of oneself as a sexual being.

Because fear of failure is high, worrisome thoughts intrude on the pleasure of sex: Have the hormones done their job? Is the timing just right for fertilization to occur? If fertilization does occur, will the fetus survive the entire pregnancy?

Any loss of sexual desire may be aggravated by the sadness and depression that are often a response to the losses incurred during the struggle with infertility. Furthermore, women who take hormonal medications may experience depression as a side effect, and the weight gain associated with these drugs may compound the depression. Few women welcome a weight gain when they are already worried about their physical attractiveness: "When we have sex, I don't feel very sexy . . . I feel deformed, physically flawed. My husband tells me nothing's different for him as far as being turned on, but I don't believe him. I feel less womanly, less sexy."

Aspects of the infertile identity thus interfere with sexuality. Feelings of being less feminine or less masculine, or of being physically defective are likely to intensify whenever the couple attempts to make love.

"Our sexual problems have been going on since we first tried to get pregnant. . . . When I couldn't get pregnant for all those months, I felt something was wrong with me. I didn't have much desire then. . . . When it turned out he was the problem, the tables turned. . . . Every time we'd try to have sex, I'd think of him as less of a man; he'd touch me, and I'd cringe."

The Effect of Medications

Hormonal medications are likely to intensify women's emotions. Many feel that they are subject to extreme mood swings and that their feelings are out of control. They feel less able to discuss their concerns, fearing they will be reduced to tears. Men may discount their partners' concerns, chalking them up to hysterics or hormones, which can leave women feeling patronized. When women express their exasperation with this attitude on the part of their partners, men often find it difficult to empathize. Inevitably, these drug-induced patterns take a toll on the couple's relationship.

The Plow and the Bridge

Infertility, as mentioned earlier, is like a plow moving through the couple's life; it unearths problems and conflicts that were partially submerged or completely buried. During Immersion, interactional patterns are likely to become more pronounced, and conflicts, typically rooted in family-of-origin histories, reemerge. As a consequence, these conflicts and problematic patterns may become more deeply entrenched, and partners may become increasingly alienated and polarized.

On the other hand, coping with the crisis of infertility can motivate couples to reexamine these old conflicts and to reshape their inter-actional patterns. Because infertility is a formidable adversary, it can force partners to forego arguments in order to act as a coordinated, empathetic, and supportive team. In this way, infertility serves as a bridge between the partners during Immersion, leading them to resolve past differences and to improve their current functioning.

THE COUPLE AND THE SUPPORT SYSTEM

Our culture offers no mourning rituals for the unique losses of infertility (e.g., menstruating when hoping for a pregnancy, pessimistic opinions of infertility specialists, miscarriages, negative lab results, failed treatment procedures, etc.), and those people closest to the couple are unlikely to understand the depth of the couple's sorrow. Thus, the grief of infertility is neither validated nor given an outlet for expression.

Family and friends, and sometimes partners, are distressed to find that seemingly minor things will hit a painful nerve and trigger an epi-sode of tears. Invariably, someone suggests that the infertility patient is being "overly sensitive," "too touchy," and "too hung up on the 'preg-nancy thing.' "

> When Renee and John finally got pregnant after several years, they slowly began to allow the idea of the baby to materialize in their minds, naming the baby-to-be Ellen. They subtly began to reorga-nize their lives and their home for the baby. Renee and John related to the fetus as if it were a baby, but, sadly, Renee miscarried. She experienced it not as a vague, nameless loss, but as the loss of the real person she had imagined Ellen to be. She wanted to share this loss with her close friends and her sister. Although she feared that others would not understand, she felt as though she would be betraying Ellen if she did not talk about her loss.

Couples are often confused and may send conflicting messages about whether they want others to respect their need for privacy or to reach toward the couple in a show of support. For this reason, friends and family become increasingly perplexed about how to respond to the couple: "My mother tells me she never knows if she should ask me about how I'm feeling or back off and say nothing," said Alice. "And, frankly, I'm never quite sure myself."

Friends and relatives may expect couples to "carry on as usual," especially as the infertility becomes "old news." They may invite the couple to family gatherings and celebrations, reasoning that the festivities will cheer up the couples and "take you out of yourself." If the partners are experiencing ongoing sadness or reacting to a recent loss, the contrast between their sadness and the festive nature of the occasion can be upsetting for everyone.

> Henry had just learned that his 8-week-old embryo no longer showed signs of life: "Could you imaging being told you should attend a 3-year-old's party 'to cheer you up' if you'd just lost a child. . . . Why can't they understand that it's just the same to me?"

Another painful experience for couples is unsolicited and unhelpful advice from others. Couples often report that close relatives or friends compare infertility to "more serious" conditions such as cancer or the "real" death of a child.

> The mother of an infertile woman tried to comfort her daughter by saying, "Snap out of this. You're healthy, you don't have cancer or anything really serious. Besides, you can always adopt."

The mother's statement is an example of the kinds of messages that are implicitly or explicitly expressed to couples in an attempt to comfort them:

- *Your distress is lasting too long.* Friends and relatives may be supportive at first, but many reach a point at which they can no longer rally any empathy
- *Infertility is not a serious medical problem.* Although infertility may be seen as a physical problem, unlike conditions such as cancer, it poses no life-threatening risks. Instead, infertility is a life-compromising condition in that it prevents one from achieving biological parenthood.
- *Adoption can be an adequate solution to infertility.* As discussed in Chapter 11, although adoption is a solution to childlessness, it is not a remedy for the losses that are experienced during infertility.

The mother's statement lacked an appreciation of how infertility makes people feel abnormal, defective, and damaged, and the critical nature of the message suggests that the feelings are excessive: "I felt like she was scolding me for being a baby, being too emotional. Somehow I wasn't reacting the way I ought to."

Although friends and relatives may have good intentions, such comments add yet another layer of distress. Unfortunately, the gap in understanding can make couples feel even more isolated from the "healthy world," a world in which they were included before the infertility surfaced.

Childlessness is not the norm in our society, and couples struggling with infertility are painfully aware of this. They may find it disturbing to be regarded as unconventional or even abnormal. Couples may be hypersensitive to how they think they are being perceived by others because they are childless: "We just want to be like everyone else, but instead we stand out."

During Immersion, many couples also contend with implicit and explicit social disapproval of their choice to seek medical treatment for infertility. Due to society's focus on overpopulation and the shortage of homes for abandoned and orphaned children, couples may feel defensive about their wish to have a genetically related child (Bartholet, 1993). Unlike fertile couples, who are rarely, if ever, challenged about having babies, couples struggling with infertility feel they are being judged as "politically incorrect": "I don't know what makes me feel worse," said Glenn, "having to deal with the infertility, or having to defend our decision to turn to medicine."

THE COUPLE AND THE MEDICAL SYSTEM

Before medicine could offer so many options for the treatment of infertility, couples who wanted children relied on the hope that conception would occur naturally. Although couples undoubtedly became emotionally preoccupied with getting pregnant, there were few proactive steps that they could take to increase fertility. Medical remedies were limited, so couples relied more on folklore than science, for example, taking to heart the erroneous advice, "Relax, and you'll get pregnant."

Dramatic shifts have taken place in the past decade; almost daily there are reports of new technologies and of medicine's victory over another obstacle to fertility. Therefore, today's couples become increasingly involved in medical treatments, as new and better techniques appear: "As soon as we think we've exhausted every possibility, the doctors break through another barrier."

Duration of Immersion

Some encounters with infertility will be limited, whereas others may drag on for years. A study by Patterson (1991) found that although some couples may devote as much as 15 years, the average time spent pursuing infertility treatments is 2–3 years. However, Patterson's research may not reflect the effects of the newer technologies on a couple's decision to remain in treatment. These effects can be twofold: Continual technological advances may increase couples' choices, therefore lengthening their involvement with medical treatment; at the same time, medical progress will continue to shorten the time spent in Immersion for many couples. New technologies and diagnostic procedures may allow physicians to diagnose and treat certain infertilities faster and with greater success. For example, ICSI, which was unavailable to couples only a few years ago, has dramatically changed the picture by offering an effective treatment for a host of male factor infertilities.

After couples have tried several cycles of a treatment protocol; invested their time, energy, and money; and endured psychological and marital distress, they often feel compelled to keep trying, believing that their efforts will eventually pay off. This may keep them in Immersion for years. Some couples use terms such as "obsessed with" or "addicted to" treatment to describe how they feel.

> With pained humor, Steve suggested that he and his wife start a group with other couples like themselves who have exhausted their bank accounts, devoted their lives to treatments, and endured enormous psychological distress while pursing the elusive goal of a baby: "We'd call it Infertility Treatments Anonymous . . . we just can't stop; we don't know how." However, when asked whether he might actually try to start such a group, he quickly backed off, saying they were not ready "*quite yet.*"

Couples who spend a relatively short time in Immersion are likely to be:

- Older couples who must race to beat the clock, attempting to conceive before the woman's age makes that impossible. Their time spent in Immersion may be relatively short but very intense.
- Couples (whether older or in their prime childbearing years) who are less invested in the idea of parenting and consequently undergo few, if any, medical procedures.
- Couples who are able to conceive a child with relatively few medical interventions soon after the diagnosis of infertility is made.
- Couples who quickly learn that one partner is totally unable to reproduce and who rule out the option of using third-party conception or other reproductive technology.
- Couples who reject medical interventions because their moral, religious, ethical, or aesthetic convictions are incompatible with

assisted reproduction. The Roman Catholic Church, for example, rejects all IUI and IVF procedures and regards workups that
involve masturbation as "morally dubious" (U.S. Office of Technology Assessment, 1988, pp. 364–368). Orthodox Judaism
regards procreation as an essential value and approves of infertility workups and treatments (with minimal use of masturbation).
However, it rejects the use of donor gametes (U.S. Office of
Technology Assessment, 1988, pp. 364–368).

Although some couples may find the medical route unsuitable,
undesirable, or unaffordable, if they strongly desire children, their hope
of having a child may extend beyond the decision to forego treatment.
Although they never enter the medical arena, having a baby remains a
dim but ever-present possibility. Neither in nor out of active Immersion,
it may be difficult for them to put closure on their hope of having a child
until the woman's childbearing years are over.

Making Medical Decisions: The Treatment Treadmill

By entering the medical arena, the couple is buoyed by the hope that this
track will lead to pregnancy. Each step into the treatment process com-
mits them further. Early decisions are often relatively easy, but in making the first choice to go ahead with treatment, the couple may be paving
the way for an automatic acquiescence to more difficult and expensive
decisions later. Physicians often recommend multiple trials of a procedure. This can put the couple on "automatic pilot" as they continue to
undergo treatment without thoroughly evaluating whether it is wise to
proceed. Because couples do have a choice, they should evaluate the following factors before proceeding: costs, success rates, side effects, the
possibility of multiple births, and psychological effects.

Costs

The costs of diagnostic and treatment procedures are high (see the
Appendix) and affect the decision to continue treatment. Fees may be
less of an issue at the beginning of Immersion when hopes are high and
funds have yet to be tapped. But as time passes and the bills for treatment accumulate, many couples exhaust their savings and may even sink
into debt. Seeing their assets shrink, they are forced to rethink the strategy of "a baby at all costs."

> "We've gone through what we put aside for a down payment on a
> house. . . . We nixed the idea of buying a safer car, and we started

withdrawing from a very small account we hoped would be the start of a college fund," said Glenn. "It makes you think, what kind of life are we going to offer this kid if he or she is ever born?"

Some couples literally "go for broke" and leave treatment only when their cash runs out: "We had to stop after we took out loans from her family and mine, and we maxed out our charge cards." Couples who exhaust their finances and end up without a baby may be left with great resentment and bitterness. Sometimes the anger is directed at the physician or medicine in general, and sometimes at themselves or each other.

Success Rates

Because the odds for success are usually factored into couples' decisions about initiating or repeating specific protocols, couples need reliable information to help them evaluate their chances for success (see the Appendix). Unfortunately, some physicians and clinics may prod couples forward with statistically skewed data that makes the couples' chances of getting pregnant seem greater than they actually are. Generally, live birth rates with infertility treatments are less than 50%, and can fall below 7% for certain ART procedures for women over age 40 with a male infertility factor (SART, 1998). Nevertheless, even with accurate information, couples may have different reactions to the possibilities of success.

> Lorraine was "thrilled" to learn that the infertility specialist thought that the probability for success in a first IVF was "as high as 15%," and she could not wait to begin treatment. The same statistics disheartened her partner, Howard, who said that "an 85% failure rate did not seem very promising." While she talked about the possibility of "winning the jackpot," he felt that the protocol was a poor investment.

Sometimes, although a physician may voice strong doubts about success or even refuse to perform any further medical interventions, couples' passionate wishes for children may lead them to ignore medical advice. Unwilling to leave the medical arena, these couples seek out doctors who are willing to proceed; some will travel great distances in pursuit of new techniques.

> One couple, who were thousands of dollars in debt, "did not waste any time thinking where the money would come from" when they heard of a "promising" new procedure in Israel; within days, the wife was on a plane to the clinic.

Side Effects

In deciding to continue treatment, couples weigh short- and long-term side effects (see the Appendix). Many surgical procedures can be physically demanding and painful. In the short term, hormonal treatment may produce mild to severe symptoms like those of PMS, as well as weight gain and the possibility of ovarian hyperstimulation (Marrs, 1997).

> "I feel so bad," said Nancy. "I'm either gaining weight or losing weight. I don't exercise. I eat badly. I'm full of anger, and I'm jumpy all of the time. I'm just one progesterone ball. I feel awful about myself; I feel inadequate. I don't want to have sex. I don't want to be touched. I don't know if we should keep moving forward, and yet I'm unable to stop."

Long-term side effects of the hormonal medication must also be considered by the couple. Although some studies suggest that the risk of ovarian cancer is small (Rossing, Daling, Weiss, Moore, & Self, 1994; Whittemore, 1994), the research remains inconclusive.

> "This is, I think, the seventh time I'm taking Perganol. . . . At first we thought the risk was insignificant considering that we could finally have a baby, and I'm still willing to go ahead with another cycle, but at some point, I think I may need to stop. I'm starting to worry more about what I might be doing to my body. . . . I hope I don't regret this later if we don't have a baby and I have physical problems."

Multiple Births

The possibility of having multiple births must be considered when deciding to continue medical treatment: The chance of multiple births in procedures in which several embryos are transferred (e.g., IVF) can be as high as 40% (SART, 1998), and, statistically, multiple births result in more medical problems than single births. In addition, if several embryos implant, couples may find that they are faced with the prospect of reduction (the surgical removal of one or more fetuses) and that the viability of the pregnancy is in jeopardy, as surgical reduction to ensure the health of the babies and mother may itself trigger spontaneous abortions. Couples may therefore face an agonizing decision in which neither alternative is acceptable.

Caring for multiples is a daunting prospect for most parents. Many who seek infertility treatments are couples in their late 30s and 40s, and these older couples may find it hard to cope with sleepless nights and active toddlers.

Regarding these complex decisions, in general, the couples with whom we work are well-informed and medically sophisticated consumers of infertility services.

> "In a sense, we have no choice, we have to be experts. . . . There [are] so many decisions to make [that] you've just got to know what it's all about. . . . I think I was deluding myself before [the infertility was diagnosed]; I ignored facts [regarding declining fertility for older women] that were out there. . . . So, I'm not going to let that happen again. . . . This time I'm going to be on top of it."

Mourning and the Medical System

Couples who have not yet experienced unsuccessful treatments may be ill-prepared for the feelings of loss that accompany failed procedures. The periodic lab results (e.g., successful or unsuccessful fertilization of an IVF procedure, positive or negative pregnancy tests, blood tests about whether a pregnancy is still viable, etc.) may be occasions to grieve, depending on success or failure. Clinic personnel, even those who try to be attentive to patients' needs, can sometimes forget this, and they may brusquely relay negative lab results in ways that can seem insensitive: "Can you imagine calling up an airline to find out if a family member was on a plane that crashed, and the airline says, 'What's the name? Oh, yeah, he's dead.' "

Some clinics seem to be less aware of both infertility's chronic distress and the grief that couples experience after learning of a treatment failure. There are also physicians who seem to know that couples experience a great deal of pain and distress, but prefer to keep the focus on the hopeful rather than upsetting aspects of infertility. This may be, in part, because these physicians think that the emotional aspects of infertility are best handled outside of the clinic environment, and many may not have the time or temperament to form empathic ties with their patients.

On the other hand, many clinic personnel are exceptionally sensitive to the patients' emotional needs and even become a temporary support system for couples who feel misunderstood by their family and friends. Clinic personnel may listen to patients' distress and take extra time comforting and supporting patients. Although this is certainly preferable, it too can have unfortunate effects.

> Evie received a great deal of reassurance, encouragement, and "cheerleading" from Suzanne, the physician's assistant. When, after a seventh treatment procedure, Evie started to menstruate, she could not bear to disappoint Suzanne, feeling it would only com-

pound her own sense of failure. Like an Olympic athlete who feels she has let her coach down, Evie was "so ashamed" that she asked her husband to place the call to the clinic.

No Time to Mourn

Whereas younger couples struggling with infertility may able to suspend treatment and take the time to mourn treatment failures, older couples who are anxious about the passage of time, their relentless adversary, often feel they have little choice but to undergo medical protocols in quick succession.

> In their early 40s, Sarah and her husband, Nat, spent little time mourning the miscarriage of a 7-week-old fetus before launching into another treatment protocol. "Grieving is a luxury," said Sarah; aware of the "closing window of opportunity," she was panicked by the idea that she might run out of time.

Therefore for older couples, unlike their younger counterparts, the time intervals between protocols are determined more by biological imperative rather than emotional readiness. It is important to add that physicians, like many of their patients, are often working against time.

> One physician told his patient that although in an ideal world she could take some time to mourn her recent miscarriage, she might be sadder, in the long run, if she let precious time run out. If she waited, his job would be that much harder, and getting pregnant might be out of the question.

> After a series of treatment failures, the incompletely mourned losses, unspoken or underexpressed sadness, disappointment, anger, and frustration accumulate. This may lead to depression, which can be quite severe, with patients sometimes experiencing suicidal thoughts (Boivan et al., 1995). One woman, who miscarried in her sixth week of an IVF-assisted pregnancy, became so depressed that she took to her bed and could not care for her 5-year-old daughter.

SECONDARY INFERTILITY

Although Rhonna was in her late 30s, she became pregnant on the first try. When her daughter was 2 years old, she and Ed decided they wanted to have a second child. This time they were unsuccessful. Ed said, "Mother Nature played a terrible trick on us in letting us get pregnant so easily the first time. We thought we were so fertile." Rhonna was angry that she had not been warned about the difficulties she might encounter by waiting: "I'm mad at my doctor, I'm mad at the women's movement, I'm mad at society, I'm mad at everyone who made me think I could get pregnant whenever I wanted. Why didn't my doctor tell me if I wanted another baby, I should get going? I thought I had endless amounts of time, and now I've blown it."

The Immersion phase can be a very difficult time for couples struggling with secondary infertility. Shock at the diagnosis of infertility is superseded by the challenge of coping with the dual demands of parenting and infertility treatments. Many women who enjoyed pregnancy and childbirth feel a sense of loss at the idea of never experiencing it again; thus, the loss for women with secondary infertility can be particularly painful. Indeed, both parents may have a bittersweet feeling of longing for another child, knowing what they might be missing.

The grief of secondary infertility is often confusing: "I have one child. What do I have to complain about?" Parents may feel sad about not having another child, but at the same time feel guilty toward the child they already have. They are often chagrined to find themselves feeling that this child is not enough.

Couples struggling with secondary infertility find few who can sympathize with their situation. People with primary infertility find it especially difficult to understand the couple's pain because the couple already has a child. On the other hand, people with more than one child may think they are comforting those with secondary infertility by saying things like "What do you want two for? All they do is fight." "Two is double the work. You want another one in diapers?" As the grief and disappointment of infertility mount, few can understand the couple's distress, and consequently the partners feel increasingly isolated. In addition, whereas couples with primary infertility can avoid child-oriented places and events, those with secondary infertility do not have that option and often are in the position of socializing with mothers who are having more children.

Existing children may ask for siblings as other friends are having baby sisters and brothers. Often, the goal of providing a sibling may come to seem more important than attending to the current needs of the child. On a practical level, the child's needs may conflict with the demands of medical treatment. On an emotional level, the parents may have little energy for the child even when they are between treatments. Furthermore, hormonal treatment and failed procedures can make it difficult to parent. Parents may worry that they are neglecting their existing child in their single-minded pursuit of a pregnancy.

Whether primary or secondary infertility, the Immersion phase is the most intense and distressing, and therefore, the phase in which couples are most likely to enter therapy.

8

⌁

THERAPEUTIC APPROACH IN THE EARLY AND MIDDLE IMMERSION PHASE

"The desire to have another child outweighs everything else that goes on for me physically and emotionally during the month I'm on my medication. And there is also the factor that we've gone this far. It's impossible to imagine stopping at this point."

PRESENTING PROBLEM

With the diagnosis of infertility and the increased involvement with the medical system, couples tend to experience heightened stress and anxiety and subsequently are most likely to come into therapy. Couples often fail to realize how profoundly their distress is affecting the marital relationship until the situation feels dire. The shifting extremes of hope and despair have a cumulative emotional effect on each partner and put great stress on the couple's relationship. Couples eventually become concerned that the marriage will no longer be able to tolerate the tribulations: "If we ever have this baby, his or her parents may be divorced." But even though many couples talk about infertility being a "make or break" ordeal for the marriage (see Chapter 5), because their motivation to get pregnant is so strong, they are willing to take the risk of psychological and relational stress.

RESPECT AND LIMIT THE POWER
OF INFERTILITY

Couples at this stage are in the grip of a devastating experience. They often encounter a degree of pain seen in families in the wake of events such as the death of a child or the diagnosis of a life-threatening illness such as cancer. The clinician needs to take this into consideration in assessing the couple, recognizing that a high level of distress on the part of each or both of the partners is common during this phase. Another aspect for the clinician to bear in mind is that hormonal medications greatly amplify a woman's emotional responses and her affect can become labile and intense. Her partner may find it increasingly difficult to cope with her distress, and the relationship may start to fray. Because of the focus on achieving pregnancy, couples may not come for therapy until their emotional problems are severe.

> Frank and Cheryl said that had they not been so focused on getting pregnant, they would have noticed the toll on their relationship much earlier. "We started to question whether we could stay together if we ever got to be parents. Then we knew we had let things go on much too long."

Some relationships have become so strained that angry feelings between partners are a subtext to most of their communication. These feelings can erupt suddenly in bitter verbal outbursts. Rather than assume that this is typical of the couple's functioning, it is more reasonable for the clinician first to assume that infertility has gotten the better of one or both members of the couple. It is helpful to block the negativity and briefly state that these kinds of outbursts are the unfortunate result of the anguish that infertility generates.

The therapist can also expect to see what may seem like extraordinary optimism. Often cultivated as a way of coping with doubts and fears about achieving a pregnancy, this optimism can seem forced and desperate. A woman may, for example, report numerous treatment failures and yet seem convinced that the next protocol is sure to succeed. A clinician with little experience treating this population may be misled into accepting the inevitability of success or, more likely, may wonder about the client's ability to assess reality accurately.

In view of the powerful effects of infertility, it is therefore best to defer any assessment of functioning and personality. Often therapy can have a dramatic stabilizing effect; by the second or third session, the couple may already seem calmer and less distressed.

THE THERAPIST'S ROLE

If the clinician has a proparenting bias, it may be difficult for him or her to accept a couple's decision to draw the line at certain procedures. On the other hand, the clinician may become intoxicated with the couple's enthusiasm, or anxious about his or her own possible infertility. He or she may feel it is inappropriate to question doctors' advice when they recommend further treatment. In such cases, he or she may find it exceedingly difficult to ask questions about the cessation of treatment or the possibility of treatment failure.

When a therapist is hesitant to introduce topics such as ending treatment or treatment failure for fear of spoiling hopeful fantasies, it is helpful to consider the relevance of raising these possibilities. Conversations with clients should include a perspective regarding where they are in the process and a consideration of their choices before they "automatically" take the next step. Clinicians can also help couples be better prepared for treatment failure. When the possibility of failure is suggested, it may open up a painful but necessary aspect of the discussion—an important component of the therapy.

The therapist should explore alternatives to a genetically related child. Some therapists may be more comfortable asking about adoption, but may avoid discussion of a life without children. It is important to mention this possibility early in Immersion. because, delaying the discussion until later may contribute to the couple feeling that the clinician endorses the prevailing belief that couples *must* have children.

> After a clinician raised the possibility of choosing a life without children if all treatment failed, John looked hesitantly at his wife, and then began to voice his feelings and thoughts about the matter. Although his wife, Renee, was opposed to such an outcome, John was able to air his side. At one point he said, "I feel so relieved just being able to talk about this with you. . . . I know we'll probably end up with a child one way or another, but I wanted Renee to hear the other side. So far, when I raise this possibility, I get the sense that people think I'm abnormal."

An important issue is the therapist's attitudes toward adoption. A couple may want either a jointly conceived child or no child at all, and may not see adoption as an acceptable consideration. In this instance, a therapist who views adoption as a viable solution may see the couple as selfish, not really committed to parenting, or too quick to give up on the chance to experience the fulfillment of parenting. However, if the clinician has a negative attitude about adoption, he or she may not fully engage a couple in discussing the reasons for rejecting this option. Subsequently, the therapist would not be providing the partners with an opportunity to sort through their beliefs about raising a child that was not a product of their genes. The couple then loses an opportunity to confront and perhaps modify those beliefs. Many couples who begin with an aversion to adoption find that it becomes more acceptable after they experience numerous treatment failures.

When the couple has strong differences regarding aspects of the treatment protocols, the therapist must recognize and set aside his or her own personal preferences. Only then can he or she be rigorous in exploring all the possibilities in order to validate fully the concerns of both partners. When appropriate, it is also important to raise other alternatives.

As in all therapy, a pitfall of treating couples facing infertility is that the clinician can easily get caught up in discussing the content to the exclusion of the process. It is important for the therapist to stay focused on the larger view, questioning each partner's beliefs, assessing whether they are in agreement regarding how to proceed. In situations where partners seem to be of one mind, it is still important for the therapist to raise alternative considerations in case one partner has conceded prematurely to the other partner's desires.

LOCATE THE COUPLE ON THE TRAJECTORY

When couples are in Immersion, they can become stuck in a limbo, existing neither as parents nor as "nonparents." It is difficult for them to retain a sense of perspective. They may feel as though the ordeal will never end and that their anguish is permanent. In early Immersion, the distress is usually combined with intense involvement in medical treatment. The couple is very busy, functioning in a problem-solving mode. By middle Immersion, the focus on treatment has often excluded social life, career, and enjoyable activities. By late Immersion, numbness and lethargy may set in. It is often helpful to remind couples that infertility is a time-limited problem, that distress is normal, and that although it may be difficult to imagine it now, they will take up their lives again in the future.

WORKING WITH THE COUPLE: THERAPEUTIC ISSUES, TECHNIQUES, AND STRATEGIES

Pacing of Sessions

The emotional and practical aspects of infertility during this phase require flexibility on the part of the clinician in the scheduling of sessions as discussed in Chapter 2. The couple can come for a session in order to process feelings about specific events; for example, coming in before an IVF transfer procedure, then not again until after hearing whether or not the embryo implanted. This flexibility allows the couple to be in charge of the agenda, which in turn gives them some control over time—a commodity often sacrificed to infertility treatments.

Speaking the Unspeakable

Separate Sessions

During Immersion, holding separate sessions can be especially helpful. The therapist might frame these meetings as a place to talk about complex feelings about the infertility. The clinician can add that during these separate sessions, partners are often helped to realize that their concerns and feelings can be shared with the other without having dire consequences and that by speaking freely, they may strengthen the couple bonds. The clinician can then encourage partners to speak about their secret fears and fantasies, and the thoughts and feelings that each believes cannot be shared with the other. The therapist can normalize these fantasies and explore how and at what cost to the relationship these may be shared or kept secret.

In the separate sessions, it is important to validate each partner's experience. In this process, the clinician can gently probe for problematic beliefs and conflictual feelings that may be contributing to the pain. Embedded in the sadness, there may be feelings of grief, anxiety, and anger. Feelings of defect, whether about the self or the partner, a sense of being less womanly, less manly, or less sexy, and fantasies of ending the relationship or having a baby with another person are common. Often, these ideas are so overwhelming that each partner feels that they cannot be discussed with the other.

An issue that frequently arises in separate sessions with men is that they feel as though they are not entitled to an equal voice in decision making about infertility treatments. They feel they can support their partner's ending treatment, but that they cannot ask her to continue with treatment because her body is the site of most procedures. As an offshoot of this thinking, they also feel that they cannot discuss their feelings of helplessness with their partners. In order to bring his voice into the couple sessions, the therapist can first normalize the man's feelings by stating that such feelings are common in these situations, and then open up the possibility of his discussing his sense of powerlessness with his partner. The idea is not so much for the man to gain an equal voice as it is for him to acknowledge his feelings.

An important intervention, when partners are reluctant to discuss significant thoughts and feelings with each other, is for the clinician to explore by asking future questions about the longer-term implications of talking or not talking to one another. We cannot overstate the power of "future questions" (Penn, 1985) and the importance of maintaining an atmosphere that allows couples to speak openly about their deepest, sometimes painful thoughts and feelings with each other.

Using Metaphors

In exploring meaning and belief systems, clients' metaphors about themselves and the infertility will often be revealed. Working with metaphors is especially helpful for couples undergoing this ordeal because metaphors help them describe their experience. Metaphors provide a means of escaping the language of dysfunction and deficiency. The therapist can help couples to liberate themselves from the verbal traps in which they get caught. In capturing experiences in less restrictive language, new options can be discovered or created. After revealing current constraining metaphors by which couples define themselves or their infertility, the clinician can then ask clients to create a related but alternative metaphor, thus reframing the material in a positive light.

> When Sid was diagnosed as being infertile, Deborah had decided to have a child using DI. In exploring their belief systems, the therapist asked, "How included or excluded will Sid feel about having a child with donor sperm?" Deborah replied, "Sid feels excluded from everything. He uses this imagery that he's a lone wolf on the tundra." The therapist asked whether Sid might be able to change the metaphor of lone wolf to a more inclusive one.
>
> At the next session, Sid had indeed re-envisioned himself: "I want to be more active, more like a guardian protector role, so I thought about being an English sheepdog whose role is to guard the sheep."

FACILITATE MOURNING

Because Immersion is the most physically demanding phase, many of the couples' losses are quite tangible such as failed treatment attempts and miscarriages. However, the grief response is not always predictable. Some, for example, regard a failed ART procedure as disappointing but not yet a loss. Others respond to each failure as though it were a major loss. Sometimes the second, third, or fourth failed attempt is the one to trigger deep sadness, perhaps because the doctor suggested that optimum success would be reached after a certain number of cycles.

> Lydia, who had moved through the process in a calm and intellectualized way with no real experience of loss, found herself uncontrollably sobbing when the doctor suggested postponing her first IVF procedure because of a medical concern. She realized her response was out of proportion to the doctor's suggestion and recognized she was responding to the accumulated and unacknowledged feelings of frustration, helplessness, and loss.

At each session, the clinician may want to track how the couple is experiencing and dealing with the losses by posing questions such as the following:

- Which one of you experienced the [treatment failure, miscarriage, etc.] as a greater loss?
- Which one of you is more inclined to speak about it with the other?
- What might be the consequences of not discussing this particular [treatment failure, miscarriage, etc.]?

Although each partner may experience their losses differently and at different times, helping them to express their feelings and feel validated is a major part of our work.

> Mary and Donald, who were proceeding with a donor sperm procedure, experienced grief at different times. For him, it hit when he was diagnosed as sterile. But the moment of extreme loss for her was at the time of conception with another man's sperm: "I didn't think anyone else would ever understand that . . . and I am not sure anyone else will, outside of this room." As part of the process, the therapist enabled Mary to articulate the actual nature of her loss.

Use of Rituals

Rituals formalize and demarcate the passages of life (Imber-Black & Roberts, 1993). They function as a vehicle by which people can make transitions between one status, relationship, pattern, or psychological state to another. As discussed in Chapter 2, they can play a crucial role in the process of grief and mourning. Although there are no established rituals for the losses of infertility, Fein (1998) reports that rituals for miscarriages are becoming common. Due to the technology that allows couples to see a fetus at a very early stage, the loss of the fetus seems more real and needs to be acknowledged and grieved. Rituals may also be appropriate for other losses such as menstruation or the inability to have a jointly conceived child.

The clinician can suggest several ideas to the couple to help them plan a ritual. According to Imber-Black and Roberts (1993), "rituals give many opportunities to highlight what is positive in the family (or couple) along with the chance to rework and change problematic interactions" (p. 84). The planning period can be very important in this regard and should be undertaken with care and attention so that both partners are involved and in agreement about the various elements of the ritual. The five elements that Imber-Black and Roberts emphasize are *preparation, people, place, participation,* and *presents.* Presents may not be an issue in a mourning ritual, but the clinician may suggest that the ritual include special items such as baby clothes or a memorial object of some sort—one couple planted three pine trees in remembrance of the three miscarriages they endured (Fein, 1998). As for people, it may be helpful for the therapist to mention the healing that is available to the partners as they grieve together. This does not preclude including other individuals in the ritual but emphasizes the couple dyad. To help couples prepare for their ritual, the clinician can ask the following questions:

- What do each of you need to say?
- What kind of preparation do you need to do?
- Who do you wish to include?
- Does this selected site work for both of you, and does it have a special meaning related to the mourning? (Imber-Black & Roberts, 1993)

EXPLORE THE RELATIONSHIP
WITH THE SUPPORT SYSTEM

Coaching Family and Friends

One way to help couples with the social isolation that is common during Immersion is to suggest that they coach their family and friends on how to offer appropriate comfort and sympathy. An excellent pamphlet is available from RESOLVE entitled *When You're Wishing for a Baby: Managing Family and Friends* (RESOLVE, 1998), which suggests that couples inform their support systems that anger and depression are common responses to the stresses of coping with infertility, and also suggests that couples may need to be clear about what sort of remarks are particularly hurtful. In addition, the therapist can guide the couple to make the following suggestions to family and friends:

Sometimes we do, and sometimes we do not want to talk about the infertility. Please try to take cues from us, and we will try to be clear about what we want. After we have a treatment failure, we want to talk about our loss. Please, just listen.

Although we realize you are trying to make us feel better by saying such things as "Don't worry, you can try again," "It's probably for the best," or "It's God's will," it feels better to hear statements like "I am sorry to hear what happened," "This must be very hard for you," or "I feel so bad for you."

During the first year, each significant event is likely to trigger strong grief reactions. For this reason, the couple might remind family and friends that grief lasts a long time. By approaching family and friends with these suggestions, the couple may strengthen existing bonds, or at least determine who in their support systems is not capable of providing appropriate support during this time.

Sometimes relatives that were not especially close before the infertility may become unexpected allies. One infertility patient, whose family had not been supportive about her prolonged sadness following a miscarriage in early pregnancy, received consolation from a cousin overseas:

Valerie's cousin Enid, who lived in Europe, had had fertility problems and had miscarried several times in the first trimester. Therefore, she understood Valerie's sorrow. When Enid gave birth to a son, she sent Valerie a note along with the birth announcement. It said that although Enid was overjoyed with her baby son and knew that Valerie would probably be pleased for her, she also wanted Valerie to know that Enid was thinking of her because she knew that Valerie might be feeling very sad "thinking about the baby that you miscarried 2 years ago." Enid went on to say that she remembered each of her miscarriages, "no matter how long ago they were," and that from time to time—"like when I get a birth announcement"—she would think sadly about each of the babies that never survived.

New Friends and RESOLVE

Couples, feeling isolated and out of step with colleagues, friends, family, and society at large, may look for new relationships and/or strengthen their ties with friends who do not have children. The helping professional can also suggest that they go to RESOLVE, a national self-help group with regional branches, in order to find a community with whom to share their experiences. Couples may find that RESOLVE meetings both validate the infertility experience and reduce their sense of isolation and deviance. Women are typically more eager to do so than are their partners. This may be related to the fact that, compared to men, women find infertility more distressing (Freeman et al., 1985). Also, women's socialization tends to make them less inhibited about reaching out to others when they feel vulnerable. Wives often encourage their spouses to accompany them to RESOLVE meetings. However, most RESOLVE chapters report that men are far less likely to attend group meetings for the purpose of sharing feelings. Instead, they are more inclined to use RESOLVE as a medical information resource. Unlike their wives, when men are the carriers of the infertility factor, they may feel embarrassed, even ashamed, to discuss their condition, rather than wanting to share their distress with others: "Jane thought I would want to talk about my infertility with men who are also infertile. . . . That was the last thing I wanted to do. . . . I'd be surprised if there really are other guys who want to discuss it."

Sometimes, however, RESOLVE can intensify a member's sense of being apart from the mainstream. As with many self-help organizations, an unfortunate consequence of the solidarity generated by membership is the polarization of the world into "us" and "them," in this instance, the fertile and the infertile. Even in this organization, it is not uncommon for other members to feel abandoned or betrayed when one member of the group gets pregnant and has a child. The happiness of becoming pregnant may be tempered by guilt for having achieved what the other members have not, and it may be impossible to remain in the group.

Secondary Infertility: Speaking with the Existing Child

Parents often ask the clinician what to say when an existing child asks, "Why aren't you having another baby?" The best answer is probably "We would like to have another child but something is not working in our bodies, and perhaps the doctors can help us fix it." It is important to let the child know, in appropriate language, that the medical procedures do not mean that a parent is sick or dying.

The clinician can caution the parents against statements such as "We love you so much, you are all we want. We do not need another child." This can backfire on two levels: First, the child may feel punished for being good because he or she is being denied a sibling. Second, if the couple manages to have another child later on, the first child may feel that perhaps the parents did not love him or her so much after all.

It is important to help couples understand that even if parents have not discussed it, and their children have not asked questions, they are probably aware of increased tension. The therapist can explain that it is helpful to the child to have an explanation for any tension, distress, or changes in routine, so that the child does not fall back on the "magical thinking" of childhood and feel that the distress is his or her fault (Simons, 1995). Grollman (1990, cited in Simons, 1995) suggests that it is important to allow a child to see the parent's sadness, as long as the parent also reassures the child that the grief will come to an end and life will eventually return to normal. It is also important to provide the child with a sense of security by sticking to regular routines as much as possible and enlisting other people to whom the child can turn.

Parents struggling with infertility may also have to cope with a child's anger and resentment when time spent focusing on the infertility deprives him or her of time with parents. As with other distresses of childhood, validating children's feelings and helping them express these feelings through play, painting, reading books, and so forth are also good ways to address this issue (Simons, 1995).

EXPLORE THE RELATIONSHIP WITH THE MEDICAL SYSTEM

Couples in Immersion typically become so eager to become pregnant that they may feel as though they are at the mercy of the medical system. Infertility clinics, which are a part of a billion-dollar industry, are eager to offer their services. In this pas de deux, couples continue in treatments, not always weighing the consequences of each of their choices. As in Mobilization, it is helpful for the clinician to be knowledgeable about the medical procedures couples are facing (see the Appendix).

> A recently graduated therapist realized that he had not ever engaged his couple in any discussions about the pros and cons of infertility protocols: "I guess my eyes just glazed over whenever they started talking about the alphabet soup of treatment."

> "It was all Greek to me," said another. "I figured that that part didn't really concern me."

By asking about possible side effects, costs, and so forth, the clinician aids couples in feeling more in control of their lives. In addition, he or she can empower clients to be assertive in their dealings with the doctors. One area where this is particularly salient is in regard to decisions about proceeding with certain treatments. By making their own decisions about whether or when to elect a protocol, couples may feel they have more control over their lives. To facilitate this, the clinician can ask questions such as the following:

- Had you considered not going ahead with the next IVF, or waiting a bit longer?
- Who is more eager to repeat the next procedure, you or your
  doctor?
- Have you decided how many protocols make sense to you, even
  though your doctor is suggesting a particular number?
- How would it feel to disagree with your doctor? Which of you
  would be more comfortable in disagreeing?
- What are the pluses and minuses of taking time off? (Medically,
  depending on the woman's age, waiting may jeopardize the possibility of pregnancy, but in terms of stresses on the relationship
  and each partner, it might be a positive step.)

It can be useful to help couples set guidelines for their involvement
in infertility treatment. Using the answers to the questions about time,
money, and emotional expenditure listed in Chapter 6, the therapist can
review couples' intentions regarding how much they originally wanted
to invest and see how these compare with the current picture.

If couples have exceeded what they originally planned in terms of
time and money, this can be an important juncture to evaluate how
much more time and money they are willing to expend. The therapist
can thereby help the couple to set limits on their expenditures and periodically review whether they are still within these bounds. When partners disagree about what their limits ought to be, or if they agree at first
but one wants to revise the plans after reaching the limit, conflict may
erupt. In other situations, one partner, usually the one less invested in a
pregnancy "at any cost," may not express his or her resentment. For
example, a man may feel coerced by his partner's state of distress, which
is only worsened when she feels that he wants to set financial obstacles
to the possibility of a baby. Therefore, in periodically revisiting the original budget and subsequent revisions, it is important that the clinician
not position him- or herself on either side in this conflict. Rather, one
can note the couple's conflict about the original plan and explore the
consequences of proceeding in either direction.

Danielle stated that if Ron did not agree to try again, she would
never forgive him. Ron retorted that if he went along with the plan
he would feel betrayed. On considering the consequences of taking
either fork in the road, neither of which seemed acceptable, they
came to a compromise; they would "move the goal line" one last
time. They were able to keep their agreement after another procedure failed. Danielle was not happy but felt that she had chosen
wisely: "We realized we can't change each other's minds, but we

want the relationship to be good, so we have to learn to compromise and keep our promises. I also realized I wanted him as much as having a baby." Ron said that although the last procedure put them in a financial hole, and he had worried that she would not keep her promise, he had a renewed respect for both her and the strength of their relationship.

END OF EARLY AND MIDDLE IMMERSION

As couples experience more treatment failures, they are faced with an option that is more complicated than it may first appear. Donor procedures, often offered by the medical profession as the next logical step in infertility treatments, have profound psychological implications, in that the child created will be genetically related to only one parent. Thus, it is important to give this issue an in-depth analysis before embarking on such a journey.

9

ᴥ

COUPLE ISSUES IN THE LATE IMMERSION PHASE: THE DONOR DECISION

> "When the doctors told me I was facing early
> menopause, they shut the door on one event, but it was
> not completely closed for me to give birth to a baby. So
> I immediately got caught up in the search for the right
> place for donor eggs."

CHARACTERISTICS OF LATE IMMERSION

For over a century, infertile couples have had the option of using donor insemination (DI), although it has been most widely used since the 1950s. From the earliest use of the procedure, the donors were mostly anonymous, and the procedure was shrouded in secrecy. In 1984, the first baby was born from a donated egg, and, although still somewhat controversial, donor egg procedures are now common practice.

Although the donor option may be presented as the next logical step following IVF, GIFT, ZIFT, or ICSI, using donor gametes represents a qualitatively different choice, with profound consequences (Scharf & Weinshel, in press). Because the child will be genetically related to only one of the partners, this treatment can be considered somewhat akin to adoption, with all the ensuing psychological complexity regarding disclosure. This complexity is compounded by the fact that partners do not share the same genetic relationship with the child, as opposed to families with either a jointly conceived or an adopted child.

When they are faced with the donor option (often presented by physicians as just another rung on the treatment ladder), couples may have been immersed in infertility treatments for some time. They may be reeling from a series of treatment failures or from the shocking news that one partner's gametes are not usable. Therefore, they may be primed to grasp at any opportunity that will provide them with the possibility of a child. However, if they rush into donor procedures without recognizing the complexities, once the child is born they may be faced with disturbing feelings about the child's genetic connection to only one parent, conflicts around disclosure, and confusion about the ensuing familial relationships.

Differences between Eggs and Sperm

One interesting aspect of the donor process is the remarkable disparity in the way sperm and eggs are perceived. Couples envision eggs and sperm as having markedly different connotations, clinical procedures involving egg and sperm donors are dissimilar, and the psychological reactions to and relationships with sperm and egg donors are also distinct. Aside from the fact that eggs and sperm contain genetic material, there is little else that these gametes have in common. One client likened the difference in value between sperm and eggs to that between lead and gold. Differences include the following:

1. *Sperm are more numerous and easily obtainable than eggs.* A man's ejaculate provides approximately 40–300 million sperm as compared to the one egg a woman produces once a month. With the help of follicle-stimulating hormones, the number of eggs produced each month can increase to as many as 20. In addition, whereas sperm and embryos can be frozen, to date only a few successful pregnancies have been achieved with frozen eggs.

2. *Egg donor procedures are physically far more invasive than DI procedures for both the donor and the recipient.* In terms of procedure, DI is vastly simpler than egg donation. DI requires no high-tech equipment and can be done in any doctor's office, although sperm donation procedures involving IVF and other ART procedures are more complicated. But, for male donors, the process is relatively quick and easy. The same cannot be

said for female donors. They go through a lengthy, disruptive cycle of hormone injections just as infertile women preparing for IVF and other ART procedures must do. Donors then undergo a painful medical procedure that, depending on the clinic, requires either anesthesia or twilight sleep for the egg retrieval. In addition, egg donors and recipients must synchronize their hormonal cycles so that the eggs can be used immediately upon retrieval.

3. *Compensation for egg donors is much higher than for sperm donors,* and compensation for donors is a somewhat controversial issue. Whereas sperm donors have historically been paid a fee, it is usually under $100 (Kolata, 1998). The amount of time and inconvenience experienced by egg donors is significantly greater than for sperm donors, and egg donors are correspondingly compensated more highly, currently receiving fees in the range of $3,000–$7,500. However, there are more couples looking for egg donations than there are donors, so with the recent doubling of rates in some clinics, concern has surfaced over whether donors will, in effect, auction off their eggs to the highest bidder ("Fertility for Sale," 1998).

4. *Sperm donation tends to involve more secrecy than egg donation.* Historically, when only sperm were used in donor protocols, couples were advised by their physicians to tell no one— neither family members, friends, pediatricians, nor, most importantly, the offspring (Walter, 1982). As in closed adoptions, secrecy about donor procedures was considered necessary. It was felt that secrecy would avert any legal problems connected to paternity and also protect the husband's sense of masculinity. Furthermore, it was argued that secrecy could prevent any bonding difficulties between the man and the child produced with donor sperm (Braverman & Corson, 1995). In the 1970s and 1980s, the husband's sperm was mixed with donor sperm, or couples were advised to go home and have sexual relations after DI, so couples could maintain the fantasy that the child was the man's offspring. Although blood tests for paternity were available then, they were unreliable, whereas today DNA testing is conclusive.

With the advent of egg donation and the greater involvement with the donor this required, a movement began that focused on making donor information more available to recipient couples (Shapiro, 1988). Due to the nature of the procedure, egg donation began and continued almost exclusively with donors who were more or less involved with the couple.

MEDICAL PROCEDURE

The first decision, in opting to use a donor, is whether to use a known or an anonymous donor. Once this choice has been made, the couple proceeds with either DI or the egg donation procedure. With DI, the woman is inseminated with the donor sperm in the doctor's office. Men may or may not be present at the actual insemination, but the husband's presence can help the couple feel more joined in the conception.

The egg donor procedure is considerably more complicated (SART, 1998). As there is a scarcity of egg donors, couples may have a wait of several months. Once a donor has been identified, the donor provides the eggs, which are then fertilized with the man's sperm and transferred to the wife through an IVF procedure (see the Appendix). Because this is such a complicated process, and timing is so critical, men may worry they will not be able to perform and produce sperm on demand.

> Frank and Cheryl, who had a history of treatment failures, had gone to extraordinary lengths to arrange an egg donation in another state. Frank, whose sperm was required for the procedure, described how anxious he was that he be able to have an erection and ejaculate. He kept thinking about how much was riding on his performance: They had put a great deal of time and effort into researching possible donors, and the procedure was costing several thousand dollars.
>
> After insemination, Frank's anxiety persisted as he awaited the test results to see whether fertilization had occurred. Cheryl was surprised at how much of his self-esteem and manhood were invested in his success. "When he found out his sperm had fertilized 13 eggs," she said (he corrected her to say, "15"), his enthusiasm was "like a runner who had just finished a marathon."

As with other ART procedures, the high probability of multiple births is a factor that must be weighed when considering the donor option. It is important for each partner to think about how he or she would handle a reduction should the infertility specialist recommend it (see also the Appendix). It is far more desirable for partners to be clear about their positions on the issue before the situation presents itself.

LOSS

For many couples, the idea that they will create children through the union of both partner's genes is a cornerstone of the relationship. When faced with the options of using donor gametes or adopting, they may question the integrity of their union. "If we cannot make a baby together," said Melanie, "maybe we shouldn't be married." Adjustment to the idea that a marriage need not be based on the creation of genetically related children requires mourning a shared vision and reevaluating other beliefs—whether openly acknowledged or unspoken—of the relational contract.

Genetic Loss

Partners who decide to use donor gametes both experience losses; however, their feelings are different. Although the experience of the partner who carries the infertility factor is more tangible, the fertile partner's losses can be just as profound.

The infertile partner must confront the fact that he or she will never be able to reproduce; there will be no child to carry forth that parent's genetic legacy.

> Despite her joy at the thought that a baby was coming, Barbara, a donor egg recipient, was also grieving the fact that she would not have a genetically related child: "I don't know why I feel sad and happy at the same time. . . . I keep saying how lucky I am to have this baby growing inside of me . . . it's a miracle . . . and then I think, 'I wish it was mine—really mine.' I'm so confused."

The fertile partner often feels grief over missing the experience of creating a child with his or her mate and of joining genetic material to create a child who has the traits of both parents. As one woman said in a session:

> "Everybody acts like I should be really happy that I have this option. Well, I'm not. I don't want it. I mean . . . we'll have a baby and I'll be happy, but I don't want to just have a baby. I want to have your baby. I can never know exactly how you feel . . . but I think I'm extremely sensitive to the kind of loss that you're experiencing . . . it was important for me you understand that I've experienced a really profound loss, too."

The couple may also be haunted by the "ghost" (Lifton, 1998) of the "real" child, the fully genetically related child they wanted to have together. They may think, "My kid would be very different than the one I have now." The "ghost" of the donor may also be present and, depending on the psychological makeup of the parents, may be relatively unimportant or may carry a great deal of meaning. It is common for people to see the need for donor gametes as a physical failing. This can be compounded in clients who already have feelings of defect, shame, and failure deriving from their personal histories. Just as negative experiences such as hurricanes, ecological disasters, and so forth lead to a higher incidence of depression and a feeling that one has lost his or her locus of control (Abbey et al., 1992), when the need for a donor is experienced as a traumatic event, these feeling are likely to ensue.

IMPACT ON THE COUPLE RELATIONSHIP

Secrecy and Protection

Because donor or surrogate options introduce a third party into the reproductive process, a psychological and relational triangle is created (Bowen, 1976). Partners' attitudes regarding donor procedures and the donor may lead to disturbing thoughts and feelings that they wish to conceal from each other. Although the donor is physically absent,[1] he or she may be psychologically present to a greater or lesser degree during insemination, pregnancy, and birth, and after the child is born. In this configuration, the partner whose genes are not used may feel like an outsider, and the relationship between the fertile partner and the donor may take on sexual connotations: "I hate to say this," said Donald, who had a child conceived with donor sperm, "but there were times during that pregnancy when I'd look at that belly and feel like a cuckold."

Some couples conceptualize sperm or eggs simply as genetic material, an impersonal component of fertilization. In this framework, the donor is considered an anonymous participant who serves only an instrumental function in the process of reproduction. The genes of the fertile partner, the prenatal environment, and the relationship with the child during the years of parenting are seen as the vital ingredients, far outweighing the donor's contribution: "It felt as though we were picking out a set of characteristics from a menu," said Mary, "not like we were picking out a person."

However, some people conceptualize the donor as an individual who has a more prominent position in the family constellation. From this perspective, couples acknowledge the personal significance of the donor as a birth parent: "It's a little like half an adoption." Although in adoption neither partner's genes are involved and, hence, as one man put it, "adoption levels the playing field," donor procedures may be preferred because one partner's genes *are* used and the woman has an opportunity to experience pregnancy and childbirth.

---

[1]In rare instances, when a known donor is used, he or she may involved throughout the entire process.

Psychological Reactions to Sperm versus Egg Donors

Reactions to donor procedures often depend on whether the gametes are sperm or eggs. Eggs tend to be perceived as passive receptacles unlike the more sexualized, "aggressive" sperm. These feelings and fantasies are related to phenomenological differences between sperm and eggs. Sperm are active and numerous; sperm "swim" actively toward the egg in order "penetrate" the zona and "enter" the egg. On the other hand, the female typically produces only one egg and although it moves from the ovary into the uterus, the egg "drops" and is then "carried" by the tissues where it "awaits" fertilization. Likewise, in standard sexual reproduction, the female anatomy functions as a "repository" in which to "receive" the ejaculate discharged after the male has "entered" her body.

Donor procedures may give rise to rudimentary fears of violation, disloyalty, or jealousy in women, whereas men may experience apprehensions regarding competition and encroachment of another male or sexual curiosity about the egg donor. Sperm and egg donor procedures elicit different sexual fantasies for each partner.

Egg Donation: An "Affair." Because the donated egg is fertilized with the male partner's sperm, many men and women compare this procedure to an affair. Women are typically more motivated to have a baby and are willing to undertake whatever procedures are necessary to achieve a pregnancy. Nonetheless, they may be stricken with feelings of shame, envy, and/or resentment when they contemplate the union of their partners' gametes with those of another woman.

> "I had this dream that he [her husband] was with this young girl . . . and I realized it was the donor. . . . I woke up and looked at my belly and thought, 'Oh my God, I'm carrying around their affair.' . . . It was weird, it took a few hours to shake the feeling."

Men may be titillated by the notion of creating a child with another woman, albeit only with her genes. The erotic fantasies touched off by their intimate association with another woman's genes may produce feelings of guilt and shame.

> "Suppose somebody put you in a room, and they said that in the next room is the woman you will have a child with, and you have never met her. That process is already started, and you haven't even seen this woman. She is breathing and living and existing in the next room and probably thinking of you. You are going to have a child together. That child will grow up and probably live

long after you. What happens to you? I mean, unless you are numb or dead, you have to be having feelings that are stirred in you, and they certainly were in me."

Alternatively, although men who fertilize donor eggs do not experience the sense of violation that women experience with DI, some men may feel exploited. Like women who receive donor sperm, men may resent their wives for obliging them to turn what is normally a natural, intimate, and sexually stimulating process into an artificially contrived arrangement:

"You know, the creation of a child is traditionally one of the most intimate things you can do, and yet this is one of the most detached things that has ever occurred in my life. This is very upsetting. . . . To me it's almost an abstraction. I've never even met this woman. I've never had a cup of coffee with her. I've never heard her voice. I mean, this is an arrangement made by fax and phone."

Sperm Donation: Violation and "Rape." Because sperm are imbued with more sexual connotations than eggs, women's reactions to DI may range from mild distaste to physical revulsion. From what we have learned from the couples in the Infertility Project, women undergoing DI sometimes perceive the insemination process as a form of sexual invasion; in extreme cases, DI, like many medical procedures, may be experienced as rape (Zolbrod, 1993): "It's kind of like rape or something to me, frankly. . . . It's almost monstrous to think of some other stranger's [child growing inside of me]. You know, it feels like it wouldn't even be mine."

Women frequently report feelings associated with sexual violation, namely shame, anger, and guilt. Related to their sense of violation are negative feelings about their partners; they may feel betrayed because the man's infertility has made the DI necessary. At the same time, women may feel that they are committing infidelity by conceiving a child with another man's sperm.

Men often feel conflicted when they agree to proceed with DI. They may feel responsible that their partners have to undergo an emotionally distressing experience that has nuances of physical violation. However, if they were to oppose DI, they would be standing in the way of their partners' desire to get pregnant and have a child. Once the decision is made to use DI and the procedure has resulted in a pregnancy, worries about bonding with the child and feelings of being less "manly" may arise. If men have no way of expressing their feelings especially to their partners, they may feel increasingly inadequate, angry, or depressed.

Guilt and Resentment

Even when loss and sadness are experienced by each partner, fertile partners may be reluctant to talk about their own sadness, fearing that to do so would further injure the already distressed infertile partners. In a similar vein, the latter may be so stricken with guilt about carrying the infertility factor that they conceal their feelings of loss, hoping to spare their partners any additional sadness. Partners may also harbor resentment toward each other. Fertile partners, for example, may be disappointed in their mates, yet feel that it would be unfair to talk about it. The carrier of the infertility factor, sensing his or her partner's resentment, may feel unjustly blamed. When such thoughts and feelings are suppressed, partners may pull away from each other and become increasingly tense or depressed.

Out of Synch

The philosophical and psychological significance of using donor gametes is a complex matter. The inequality in the genetic relationship with the child, the sexual aspect of the donor's involvement, the extraordinary phenomenon of conceiving a child with an anonymous donor in a high-tech setting—all these factors are present when the donor decision is weighed. Understandably, each partner may require a different amount of time to explore, evaluate, and assimilate these factors. For example, one person may be overwhelmed by all the implications of a donor procedure, while the other is eager to proceed with having the child. Such a couple, especially when under the pressure of the biological clock, can easily become polarized.

> When Mia and Tom realized that gamete donation was their only option, Mia became very enthusiastic. Despite the fact that Tom's motivation to have a child was just as strong, he tried to slow the process down. The more he raised doubts, the more she lobbied for using a donor. The intensity of their struggle made a dialogue nearly impossible. Because donor eggs were in question, Mia felt that Tom was holding his sperm hostage.

There are instances in which the couple's conflict centers around the fertile partner's refusal to relinquish the ability to have a genetically related child. The carrier may advocate for adoption whereas the noncarrier wants to use a donor so that his or her genes are passed on to the child. This is an emotionally charged issue and can lead to a great deal of conflict between partners, especially if the fertile one pressures his or her partner to use donor gametes.

Although Kevin and Suzette had looked at lists of donors provided by a sperm bank, Kevin thought they were just "window shopping" when they perused the catalogs at a sperm bank. After Suzette got pregnant through DI without informing him of her plans, Kevin was shocked and resentful. This led to problems years later.

THE INFERTILE IDENTITY

"Impostors"

Larry, whose wife conceived using donor sperm, said, "When we said Vivian was pregnant, her family came over to me and slapped me on the back, and said 'Good job,' and all that kind of stuff. I felt myself shrink inside; I felt like a big fake, I wanted out of there. . . . This is only the beginning. It's going to happen again and again, I know it."

Many couples who achieve pregnancy through advanced infertility treatments may feel fraudulent, as though they have somehow "cheated" by arriving at their pregnancy via unorthodox means, and they may retain the infertile identity, the sense that they are flawed or defective. This reaction can be greatly amplified when donor protocols are involved. In these instances, one or both partners (most often the one whose genes were not used) may be overwhelmed with the sense of being an impostor.

Dennis was touring the hospital where his baby, conceived using donor sperm, would be born: "There are certain times that it kind of comes back to me, and from my perspective I feel inauthentic, that I'll be in a situation and I'll think people can tell that we used donor sperm."

Gender Differences

The Carrier of the Infertility

In general, infertility does not affect women's feelings of sexual potency as strongly as it does men's. Women's sexuality tends not to be inextricably entwined with their fertility. Women may experience the infertile identity in other ways—not feeling feminine, feeling that they are not achieving adult status or that they are defective. In men, the evolutionary drive or culturally defined imperative to procreate links fertility and masculinity: Men often equate personal power with virility. Thus, the failure implied by the use of donor sperm is often difficult for men to tolerate: "The thought of her being pregnant with another man's sperm makes me ill," said Frank. At the very least, men may need time to adjust to and integrate an altered sense of themselves as men. When sperm donors are used, women may set aside their own distress in deference to the perceived humiliation and grief of their partners:

> "Society has told me in so many words—society being parents, friends, whatever—that Sid's loss was really the tragedy. . . . I mean, people have even told me not to cry in front of him because it will make him feel guilty."

THE COUPLE WITH THE SUPPORT SYSTEM

Disclosure

Although the decision of whether and whom to tell might be considered just one of many facets of the donor option, it is a crucial matter for the future of the couple and the child. Issues of secrecy and privacy are raised whenever children who are not genetically related to both parents are brought into a family (Schaffer & Diamond, 1993). Partners who consider donor procedures must decide whether to keep the fact of donor gametes a secret or disclose it to (1) the child; (2) members of each of their families of origin; and (3) friends, acquaintances, and strangers. Ideally, couples should make these decisions prior to going ahead with a donor procedure. Unfortunately, in their haste to get pregnant, they may not sufficiently discuss these issues. Couples who assume that lingering questions will be settled at a later time may be creating problems in the future.

Future Developments

The social, psychological, legal, and ethical ramifications of donor procedures are still being discovered. There are concerns for the welfare of those involved in the process—the offspring, the parents, the donor, and the extended families of all the parties. As donor offspring mature, many begin to search for and form relationships with their genetic parents. An article in *The New York Times* described young adults who were trying to track down the anonymous donors whose sperm was used in their conception (Orenstein, 1995). In addition, Donor's Offspring, a self-help organization has been established to assist donor offspring in finding the identity of the donors.

In cases of surrogacy (see section "Surrogacy and Gestational Surrogacy" below; also the Appendix), when the surrogate is also the egg donor, couples must be prepared to face an uncertain legal future regarding visitation and maternity rights for the surrogates. Many states have outlawed surrogacy, and others have made no legal rulings on this issue. The courts have begun to rule in disputes over custody in such cases, but, although attorneys may draw up detailed contracts regarding maternity, there is no guarantee that these will not be overturned in future legal decisions.

Postnatal Reactions

Couples may experience uncomfortable moments with their friends and relatives after the donor baby is born. Typically, when a baby is born, everyone is eager to discover a resemblance to the family. In the case of a jointly conceived child, if the child does not look like one parent, that parent may feel a little disappointed. If the child looks like neither parent, jokes may even be made about the paternity of the child. However, with a donor-conceived baby, the lack of resemblance to the non-genetically related parent may leave that parent feeling like an outsider.

THE RELATIONSHIP WITH THE CHILD

Bonding and Attachment

Bonding during pregnancy and in the immediate postnatal period is anticipated as a joyful experience, as is the attachment that will develop as the child grows. Society in general, and the medical profession in particular, may assume that the parents' attachment to a baby conceived with donor gametes will be the same as with a fully genetically related child, regardless of the donor involvement. However, when partners regret being unable to create a child together or when they have disturbing thoughts about the donor, the pleasures of bonding to the child may be disrupted. In these situations it is important to recognize that parents can have mixed feelings.

Because donor procedures are so unique, clients are often perturbed by the strangeness of conceiving in this way. However, as the pregnancy progresses, and the fetus becomes increasingly viable, those feelings are likely to fade. Nonetheless, some continue to feel a lack of connection with the growing baby.

Barbara, 7 months pregnant with twins from donated eggs, described her feelings: "I feel very detached in a lot of ways. I mean, we went through a very upsetting weekend because we gave our dog away and I feel I have nothing to show for this. We did it in anticipation of the children, but they're not here yet. Nick says they are—they kick, they're large little people at this point. But I just don't think that way. They're an abstraction to me. I haven't bonded with them yet. I feel like the twins are somehow responsible for all this pain, for us having to give our dog up for something that's just an anticipation."

Issues of attachment may differ depending on whether the donated gametes were eggs or sperm. Men may have a difficult time attaching to children conceived with donor sperm. Interestingly, Zolbrod (1993) found that men who had closer attachments with their own fathers tended to experience more feelings of loss in donor sperm situations, but also had more genuine internalized motivation to father a child.

The gender of the baby also may affect postnatal attachment, but not in any predictable way. What appears to be most relevant is the particular emotional makeup of the parents involved, as well as their family histories. Two fathers of children conceived with donor sperm illustrate this point:

Kevin was very relieved that the baby was a girl. He felt that if there had been "a little manifestation of the donor" running around, he would have had an even harder time making a connection. On the other hand, Bruce was glad to have a son because he felt that as a father he could do things with a boy, such as play baseball and go fishing, that he would not do with a girl. Without those activities, he speculated that he might have felt very removed from a daughter. In his family, men and their sons bonded around sports, whereas father–daughter relationships were more remote.

Parental Status

When donor gametes have been used, there can be a tendency to misunderstand both the normal developmental phases and the relational dynamics of family life. For example, it is a common experience in families for a child to feel closer to one parent at particular times, whether the child is genetically related to both parents, only to one, or to neither, as in adoption. However, in a donor situation, if the non-genetically related parent is not as involved with the child as the genetically related parent, the couple may attribute this to the lack of genetic ties rather than to the normal variations of attachment.

Frank and Cheryl married when they were both in their late 30s, and they immediately began trying to conceive. When she was diagnosed with early menopause, they were able to have a baby using donated eggs. Cheryl, who had been raised by an aloof and distant mother, had a poor maternal role model and initially found it difficult to attach to her son, Matthew. In time, she was able to overcome her difficulties and had a very warm relationship with the toddler. However, whenever Matthew showed a preference for his father, Cheryl was quick to interpret this as Matthew's rejection of her because she was not "really" his mother.

Similarly, in the first few months of Matthew's life, when Frank noticed Cheryl's difficulties getting close to Matthew, he interpreted this as coldness and rejection. These problems were exacerbated by the fact that Frank would tend to refer to Matthew as "my son." This phrasing was painful for Cheryl to hear: "Each time he says 'my son,' it reminds me that I'm not his biological mother." Whenever Cheryl was reminded of this fact, she tended to pull away from Matthew.

Alternatively, in order to overcome the absence of a genetic tie, the carrier of the infertility may compensate by working especially hard to form a strong connection to the child. In some instances, when donated eggs have been used, men may feel that women are so determined to attach to their children, and thereby compensate for the lack of genetic relatedness, that the men feel there is no room for them.

Jessica and Bob had healthy twin boys using donated eggs. Jessica was particularly determined to bond with the infants. She described it vividly: "If I had my own eggs, would I be so fierce about getting part of me into them? I guess at times I am obsessed with breast feeding." One unfortunate result of this was that Jessica resented Bob's participation in caring for the babies. She constantly criticized him about how he held and played with them. She wanted to claim them solely as her own and exclude him.

If the couple's relationship becomes adversarial, differences in parental status may also be used as ammunition between the partners.

Barbara, a donor egg recipient, spoke about another couple with donor-conceived children and serious marital problems. During the middle of a fight the husband threatened that if they got divorced he would get the kids because they were his. Barbara felt that was an unforgivable and unforgettable comment.

In divorce cases involving couples who used donated sperm, the courts have ruled that both parents have legal rights to the child (New York State Task Force on Life and the Law, 1998). However, with egg donor situations, the legal ramifications are just beginning to unfold.

THE COUPLE WITH THE MEDICAL SYSTEM

The couple is especially dependent on the medical system during Late Immersion. This is particularly true with egg donation because in most instances, ART is used, and the clinic provides the donor.

Anonymous versus Designated Donors

Once a couple has decided on the donor option, there are several subsequent choices to be made. The first is whether the gametes will be from a designated or an anonymous donor. *Anonymous donors* are defined as those who were not previously known to the couple, although they may subsequently form a relationship with the couple and the offspring. *Designated donors* are previously known to the couple and may include brothers, sisters, parents, other relatives, or friends of the couple. The psychological and relational issues that are raised with a designated donor are complex and may be far more variable and idiosyncratic than when using an anonymous donor, depending on the nature of the preexisting relationships between the donor and the couple. Couples may initially find the idea of a designated donor appealing because their child will not be the offspring of a stranger but will carry on the family's genetic line.

> One couple, Jennifer and James, were distant relatives, and came from wealthy, "blue-blooded" families. In a previous marriage, James had contracted a childhood disease that prevented him from producing sperm. Jennifer and James decided that they wanted to continue their lineage by conceiving with family genes. They put out the word among their extended family and were pleased when a distant cousin volunteered to donate sperm.

But as couples begin to weigh all of the ramifications of using a designated donor, many become dubious about a conception with so many difficulties, both predictable and unpredictable. Familial donations create complex role and relational dilemmas, and evoke a variety of disquieting feelings. For example, a sister who donates her eggs may feel like both an aunt and a parent in relation to the child, and like a sister-in-law and a mate in relation to the child's father. She may wish to exert proprietary rights of parenthood in relation to the child, or she may feel obligated to be more involved with the child than she would like. Another possibility involves a donor who is restrained in relation to the child, so as not to appear intrusive, whereas he or she might otherwise be much more involved.

In one family in which a sister provided the couple with her eggs, the mother lived with a constant fear that as the child matured and learned about the source of her genes, the child would abandon her for the genetically related aunt.

The gender of the known donor is also a significant factor. Sperm tends to have more sexually explicit connotations than eggs; thus, receiving sperm from family members may evoke feelings of incest.

Lou's father and brother both offered to donate sperm, but Felicia was repulsed by the "incestuous" aspect of using either man's sperm. However, Felicia said that if she had been infertile, she would not have had a problem using her sister's eggs because they bore none of the sexual connotations that sperm do.

In situations in which couples receive gametes from a relative who is part of the couple's social network, other difficulties may arise.

After Phoebe gave birth to a child conceived with her sister Amanda's egg and her husband Jim's sperm, Phoebe felt as though Jim and Amanda were joined in a way they had not been prior to the procedure. Not only did Amanda seem too closely involved in raising the baby, but Phoebe also sensed a "certain sexual vibration" between Amanda and Jim. As might be expected, before this was resolved, there were tensions in the couple's and sisters' relationships.

Choosing a Clinic

Once the partners have chosen to use an anonymous donor, they will find that clinics vary considerably in how much information they choose to make available. At one end of the spectrum are clinics whose policies are to provide couples with limited information such as the donor's physical characteristics, medical history, race, religion, education, occupation, and interests. No names are exchanged, and all other identifying information is kept strictly confidential. This approach is generally used by sperm banks and some egg donor programs.

At the other end of the spectrum are clinics, usually donor egg programs, that encourage more openness. They may provide detailed information about the donors, including photographs and their handwritten application. The recipients may also be invited to meet with the egg donor face to face. Couples may wish to do this, so that when the child gets old enough to wonder about the donor, the parents can describe her and answer some of their child's questions.

One outcome of a more open sharing of donor information is the possibility of a continuing relationship with the donor. As in open adoption (see Chapters 11 and 12), this can be beneficial for the child if he or she becomes interested in meeting the other genetic parent. Although open adoption experiences may shed some light on open donor situations, it is too soon to know how significant the similarities and differences may be.

Another case to be made for a more open approach is that couples may decide later that they want to have another baby from the same donor. Whereas it is possible to bank sperm, an anonymous egg donor may be difficult to track down. Alternatively, because fertilized embryos can be frozen (cryopreserved), couples wanting another child may have these embryos kept for them as long as they are willing to pay the monthly storage fees.

> Each time the bill for the banked embryos at the cryopreservation lab arrived, Michael and Evie were faced with the choice of proceeding with another embryo transfer. After 2 years, they suffered an enormous emotional conflict. On the one hand, they did not think that as parents in their 40s, they were able to handle a larger family (their original donor procedure produced twins). Yet, the idea of stopping the payments and thereby destroying the embryos—"pulling the plug"—seemed equally unacceptable. Although they ended up paying the bill and deferring the decision for another 6 months, they knew that they would eventually make the decision to stop payments.

Surrogacy and Gestational Surrogacy

Surrogacy and gestational surrogacy[2] are the least utilized and most controversial protocols. Of all of the new reproductive techniques, surrogacy introduces the most complicated and perplexing set of concerns for the couple and society because it separates genetics, gestation, and parenting.

Surrogacy and gestational surrogacy can be particularly distressing for couples because they have so little control over the actions of the surrogate or gestational carrier. She provides the fetal environment and has total control over the fetus in spite of any disagreements with the couple

---

[2]A surrogate is inseminated with the husband's sperm, carries the fetus to term, and at birth relinquishes the child to the couple. A gestational surrogate or carrier is implanted with fertilized embryos using the husband's sperm and wife's egg(s), or with embryos generated with donor material other than that of the gestational carrier (e.g., sperm of recipient's husband and donor egg).

over how to handle the pregnancy. She can refuse certain medical procedures against the wishes of the couple who is paying for her services. The surrogate might continue to eat poorly, smoke, drink, and use drugs, any of which might harm the developing fetus. Therefore, the couple has no ultimate control over the prenatal care that the child receives. In cases in which more than two embryos survive the transfer, the surrogate or gestational carrier might be opposed to a reduction (thereby increasing the risk to the fetuses).

SECONDARY INFERTILITY

Couples who have been able to conceive a genetically related child, and are then faced with the option of using donor gametes for a subsequent child, confront a special set of issues. Because the children will have different genetic relationships with their parents, there are concerns as to how all of the familial relationships will be affected. For example, will sibling rivalries be played out in terms of genetics? Alternatively, will parental disputes related to favoritism of one child over another involve genetic status? Clearly, these parents have a lot to consider, and they may reject the donor option altogether, choosing adoption instead. Families that include children genetically related to both and to only one parent, will face complex challenges. These families' stories are now evolving, and we will await the telling at a future date.

The donor decision involves complex psychosocial issues. Therapy with couples who have used donors will be discussed in the next chapter.

10

⤚⟳

THERAPEUTIC APPROACH IN THE LATE IMMERSION PHASE: THE DONOR DECISION

"I knew I was going to feel deprived not experiencing pregnancy and childbirth . . . but I also felt it wasn't fair to George if I went for donor sperm. . . . He might always feel like 'odd man out' because I would have a deeper connection with the child than he would."

PRESENTING PROBLEM

Some couples enter therapy around the issue of donor procedures; however, it is more likely that they will first come in during early and middle Immersion, and then later, face the donor decision. Although some infertility clinics offer a counseling session regarding donor conception, these usually do not probe for major conflicts. In addition, couples often self-censor in these sessions; they are afraid to express any ambivalence for fear that the interviewer will deny them the donor gametes.

It is unfortunate that more couples do not go to therapy to discuss donor issues. The decision is so fraught with significance that couples may regret not having spent more time considering this option. A consultation or a few sessions could help a couple sort through some of the immediate issues and consider what lies ahead. Otherwise, couples may enter therapy in the Legacy phase with marital problems or difficulties with the child. However, they may not attribute the problems to the donor conception, having never explored their own feelings about using a donor and how that might be affecting their relationship with each other and their child.

For couples who seek therapy around the donor issue, a few concerns may be prominent. They may be out of synch regarding whether or not to use a donor, and if so, whether to use a designated or an anonymous donor. Other couples seek therapy during pregnancy to discuss issues such as disclosure and the unbalanced genetic relationship with their child.

Many of the treatment issues that arise in Immersion continue into Late Immersion. Donor procedures add their own complications because of the use of another person's genetic material. It is important for the therapist to acknowledge the choices that are available through new reproductive technology. In this way, the therapist can alleviate some of the anxiety couples may feel about engaging in these relatively new techniques. A statement to the effect that "Some couples find it difficult to consider having a child in this way" provides an opening for couples to explore their own thoughts and feelings on this subject.

THE THERAPIST'S ROLE

Although there can be ethical, moral, and religious dilemmas for therapists in all phases of the infertility process, in Late Immersion the therapist's own beliefs focus on the choices couples face when deciding to proceed with a donor, and the possible psychological and relational consequences both in the short- and long-term. Therapists may have reservations regarding ART and donor conception. Some question whether using ART is morally acceptable; some object to disrupting the "natural" order of reproductive events; and some believe that the money would be better spent in adopting and providing for an orphaned child. Clinicians can have concerns about the impact of the complex donor relationships on the family and child, and the medical and emotional impact on the donor. Therapists may find particular ART or donor treatments unacceptable, such as reduction, which can be associated with an abortion, or cryopreservation.

Consequently, some therapists may find themselves in conflict with the couple's decision and may choose to disqualify themselves from working with the couple, fearing their strong beliefs could interfere with the therapy. In these situations, the therapist might make his or her beliefs explicit at the outset, and give the couple a choice of working together or with someone else.

Clinicians may find it difficult to advise couples, given the lack of research regarding the long-term outcome of donor procedures. Although DI has been in use for a century, the process was cloaked in secrecy. It was only with the advent of egg donation in 1984 that research began to explore the effects of using donor gametes on family relationships and the implications of choosing to disclose or conceal the child's origins. The therapist cannot tell the couple what is likely to happen to the child, whether or not the child will want to know about the donor, and what the repercussions may be either way. Therefore, the clinician must feel comfortable proceeding, along with the couple, into the brave new world of technology. Essentially, therapists and clients are pioneers in this field.

Even when therapists are well informed about ART or donor procedures, hearing the couple's experience and the intensity of their emotional reaction can be unsettling. While it is important to monitor one's own feelings and reactions, clinicians need to be mindful to explore the meaning these procedures have for their clients. For example, if a woman had experienced DI as a violation, the therapist might ask if the meaning of this experience has changed for her, now that she is a mother and not just pregnant.

The helping professional faces many of the issues of early Immersion regarding his or her reluctance to ask difficult questions. There may be a strong desire to collude with and thereby protect the couple by acting as though there is no difference between a donor-conceived child and a jointly conceived one. Couples are often very excited that they will finally succeed in having a baby, and the medical system generally encourages them to forge ahead, without paying attention to feelings that are likely to arise. Not wanting to dampen their enthusiasm, therapists may be reluctant to mention possible problems that might ensue. It is easy to get caught up in the momentum of the donor process and avoid asking the difficult and important questions. Yet, knowing how essential it is for couples to discuss all the ramifications of their decision to use a donor, the therapist might say, "I know how excited you are by this wonderful possibility, and I share your excitement. At some point though, it is important to discuss some of the issues around raising a child that is genetically related to only one of you, and the donor's role in the future of your family. Does now seem like a good time, or would you prefer to discuss it another time?"

WORKING WITH THE COUPLE: THERAPEUTIC ISSUES, TECHNIQUES, AND STRATEGIES

Electing to conceive with a sperm or egg donor can have profound implications for a couple's relationship. If the partners choose to have a child who is genetically related to only one of them, they must grapple with the future consequences of this disparity. It is preferable for them to consider such consequences carefully before the decision is made.

Some couples, however, may be so distressed by previous treatment failures and the prospect of infertility that they are reluctant to question any aspects of using a donor. In these situations it is important for the clinician to raise difficult issues that couples may not have fully considered. The therapist might ask the following:

- Have you each thought about the fact that one of you will have a genetic relationship with your child and one of you will not?
- How do you each think this disparity will affect your relationship with your child? Your child's feelings toward each of you? Your relationship to each other?

Bill and Daphne agreed to proceed with an adoption rather than use a donor because they did not want an imbalance in their genetic relationship to the child. Bill jokingly said, "In the middle of the night, when the baby is crying, I don't want her to say, 'Get up and take care of *your* child!' "

Some partners may put premature closure on the donor option in order to protect their spouse. For instance, the fertile partner may believe it would be too difficult for the infertile partner to parent a child to whom he or she is not genetically related. Or, for the sake of the relationship, a fertile partner may prematurely agree to adoption, feeling too guilty to refuse the infertile partner equal parental status. In other couple relationships, an infertile partner might agree to proceed with donor conception rather than prevent a fertile partner from having a genetically related child.

By slowing down the process and encouraging partners to keep talking to each other about their thoughts and feelings, the therapist enables a partner who is not ready to proceed to voice his or her doubts. Sometimes this may entail raising difficult questions.

- Is it wise to make a decision if your partner still has reservations?
- What do each of you think the consequences might be?
- What are the risks and advantages of waiting or proceeding?

Speaking the Unspeakable

The possibility of using a donor may give rise to disturbing thoughts and feelings, such as guilt, resentment, and fantasies about the donor. It is important to encourage partners to express their thoughts and feelings to each other. The following questions can be used as a starting point:

- How do you think you will feel carrying an embryo that is the combination of your husband's sperm and another woman's egg?
- How do you think you will feel having your wife pregnant with another man's sperm?
- How do you think you will feel being inseminated with another man's sperm?
- How do you imagine you will deal with these possibilities as a couple?

EXPLORE COUPLES' BELIEF SYSTEMS

The Question of Bonding: Alienation versus Attachment

Although it is expected that bonding begins in pregnancy, in donor pregnancy, with all its complexity, bonding may not occur until late in the pregnancy or after the birth of the baby: "There were times when it felt like a stranger was growing inside of me. . . . When I first started nursing, I felt like I was nursing someone else's baby . . . but that feeling didn't last long."

One concern with DI is that the man, because he is not participating in the conception, may have difficulty bonding with the child. To facilitate this connection, the therapist can encourage the man to be present at the inseminations. His presence and support of his partner at this crucial moment provide a foundation for an attachment to the child as well as strengthening the couple relationship.

Early in the pregnancy, the therapist may feel comfortable exploring the couple's feelings of alienation from the fetus, but as the fetus becomes viable, clinicians often find their own loyalties shifting from the parents to the child-to-be. If an inability to bond with the fetus is intense and unchanging as the pregnancy advances, the clinician may need to intervene. This requires a degree of finesse so that the couple feels that the therapist is attuned to the range of their feelings. His or her stance can be one in which an attachment is fostered by helping the couple to acknowledge that having a child genetically related to one parent is not the same as having a child genetically related to both. While validating the inequality of the process of donor conception, one can help the parents see the consequences of not attaching to the child by asking future questions:

- Are there any benefits to remaining emotionally disconnected from the fetus?
- If you continue to feel disconnected, how do you think it will affect parenting for you and for the child?
- What do you imagine the impact will be on your relationship if one of you remains feeling disconnected from the child?
- If you decide it is important to begin to attach to the fetus, what could you do to facilitate this?

There are multiple factors that can interfere with the bonding process, particularly unfinished intergenerational struggles.

Barbara was several months into her pregnancy and was still feeling distant from her developing twins. Although early in the pregnancy she had been distressed about carrying another woman's babies, this feeling was now less disturbing. Instead, Barbara's burning and worrisome question became "What will we tell the children?" Instead of thinking about the story of their birth, she thought of "the secret" and the implied shame of her infertility. Indeed, on further exploration, the therapist discovered that Barbara felt deep shame about the years she had lost in a substance-abusing past, which contributed to her late marriage and consequent infertility.

The problem in bonding was connected to very particular historical and psychological issues, which were in turn linked to family-of-origin legacies regarding motherhood. Although the disturbance was triggered by the use of donor eggs, its resolution lay in working with Barbara on her past and current feelings and thoughts about herself. Furthermore, in this instance, it seemed that the donor conception precipitated an early and intense focus on bonding. It is possible she may have encountered similar issues no matter what genetic relationship she had to her children. Fortunately, in the course of couple therapy she was able to do preventive work that enabled her to develop a strong attachment to her twins.

FACILITATE MOURNING

Recognizing and mourning losses can be difficult for couples in late Immersion because they are so focused on the possibility of having a child. Although using donor gametes constitutes a loss for each partner, the losses may be different and do not necessarily coincide.

Conflicts can be compounded when one partner discounts the

other's suffering (e.g., the carrier does not recognize the fertile partner's loss). In addition, they each may have disquieting thoughts about the child they might have had. These issues may be very difficult for partners to raise with one another and may be best approached during separate sessions. If partners do not feel comfortable with their distressing thoughts and feelings, and/or are concerned about talking to their partners about them, future difficulties may arise. Whether clients are seen individually or together, the following questions may help the therapist probe these areas:

- What is it like for each of you to know you are not going to have a child that you create together?
- What is it like for each of you not to have the child you imagined?
- Even though you are feeling optimistic because you are pregnant, have you each considered that you may experience feelings of loss in spite of this outcome? (This can be a particularly difficult question to put to clients when they have a viable pregnancy, but prepares them early on for the sadness that may surface later.)
- Are these issues hard to discuss with your partner?
- What are you likely to do with these thoughts? Keep them to yourself? On what occasion would you share them with your partner?
- Do you feel it is okay to have these feelings?
- What kinds of circumstances do you imagine will cause feelings of loss to reemerge for each of you?

EXPLORE RELATIONSHIP WITH SUPPORT SYSTEM AND CHILD

Disclosure to the Child

Perhaps the most important decision the couple must make is whether to tell the child about the donor. The impact on the child of secrecy versus disclosure in donor situations has not, to date, been the subject of much research. However, if the literature regarding secrecy in adoption (Imber-Black, 1993) can be applied to donor children, then disclosure in and of itself is not problematic, whereas secrecy is. In revisiting Karpel's (1980) concept that the decision to disclose information should be based on the "relevance of the information for the unaware" (p. 298), it follows, then, that the child has a right to know relevant information about his or her origins.

Lifton (1998) refers to the abiding presence of the "ghost" of the birth parents in adoption; this concept may also pertain in families with a donor-conceived child. Couples need to know that if the donor is never mentioned, the child is very likely to sense an air of secrecy (Schaffer & Diamond, 1993). The clinician can point out that secrets about a donor can be difficult to maintain, especially at important life cycle events such as birthdays or graduations, if medical problems arise, or when the donor child has a child of his or her own. Alternatively, problems may also arise when couples constantly talk about the donor; as in adoption, the child may perceive this as the parents' wish to distance themselves from him or her. However, couples may find relief in the knowledge that because donor conception does not involve the child's relinquishment by the birth parent(s), as do adopted children, they are unlikely to have the sense of rejection that adopted children can experience.

Because the use of egg donors and openness about donor conception is relatively new, couples often worry about the reaction their children will receive as they proudly announce to their peers the story of their origins. In addition, the infertile partner may be worried about the child's connection to him or her in the absence of a genetic link. In such instances, the therapist can help the parent to see that it is the quality of the parental relationship, not the genetic link, that determines the nature of the bond. Once this is grasped, the telling becomes infinitely easier.

Once couples have decided to tell the child, they will want to consider when and how to do so (see Chapter 14 for a full discussion of disclosure to the child). The timing of disclosure with donor-conceived children may depend partially on how open couples plan to be with others in their lives. If they only wish to tell the child, they may need to wait until he or she is old enough to be discreet. There are drawbacks to this approach: If parents wait too long, it can impart an air of secrecy and shame to the fact of the donor involvement. However, if parents choose to tell a young child, they have no control over the disclosure of the information. As in adoption, telling a child at an earlier age allows him or her to grow into the information, with parents embellishing the birth story with age-appropriate details as time goes on.

Disclosure to Support Systems

In addition to discussing disclosure to the child, the therapist should help couples consider whom else, if anyone, they wish to tell about the donor. If they plan to tell the child at a young age, they have more freedom about whom they choose to tell because they will not be concerned about keeping secrets from their child. However, the clinician can advise couples that if they discuss the donor option with their entire network of family and friends, they may wish that they had been more discreet once the baby is born. The following example illustrates the repercussions that may result from neglecting to consider the situation carefully. Sid and Deborah were very open about their experiences in infertility treatment, and about their choice to use donor insemination. In addition, they had been eager to be interviewed for a major magazine, which included their photograph along with their story. However, after their daughter was born, they regretted having forfeited their privacy. After people began referring to "the cute donor baby," Sid and Deborah became concerned about the effects this would have on their child. Although they were willing to be interviewed prior to giving birth, once their daughter was born they declined a follow-up interview.

Couples who want privacy may tell only their child. In so doing, by drawing a tight boundary around the information, they are limiting access to a support system. It may be helpful for them to establish a small, alternative network of trusted friends, select family members, or other families with donor children. In evaluating whom to tell, couples may want to consider whether knowledge of the child's conception is likely to affect the way people view their family.

> Arnold and Anita, who conceived using donor eggs, decided to tell only Arnold's parents, because they were concerned that Anita's parents would show favoritism toward their other grandchildren.

Disclosure with Surrogacy

The issue of disclosure is further complicated in cases of gestational surrogacy. Because the child has no genetic link to the gestational carrier, parents may feel that disclosure is unnecessary. However, Lifton (1998) believes that both a surrogate and a gestational carrier should be known to the child. First, in these "Kodak moment" times, a child may wonder why the family has no pictures of his or her mother while pregnant. Second, in the case of adoption, children often want to know who carried them for the 9 months of pregnancy (Lifton, 1998). Although this may be tied to the child's curiosity about a genetically linked birth mother, it may be that some children born to gestational carriers will want to know about the women who bore them. Lastly, because there was more than one woman involved in the child's conception, he or she may be especially curious about all of the circumstances of his or her birth.

EXPLORE THE RELATIONSHIP
WITH THE MEDICAL SYSTEM

Some couples, by the time they face the donor option, have been deeply involved in Immersion and have experienced numerous treatment failures. They may be stuck on the treatment treadmill, moving from one procedure to the next without taking time to consider the consequences of each step.

In addition to helping couples sort through the psychological implications of donor conception, therapists can assist them in negotiating the array of complex choices. One such issue is the choice between using an anonymous (unknown) versus a designated (known) donor. If a couple is contemplating using a known donor, the clinician can help them consider the possible ramifications regarding the donor's relationship with their child and with them.

END OF IMMERSION

The transition between Immersion and Resolution is a gradual one, with couples moving, sometimes imperceptibly, from being deeply involved with finding a medical solution to considering the decision to end all treatment. Many grow weary, feeling that they have faced enough disappointment and need to move on with their lives. The process is often long, and couples may continue medical treatment, with increasingly less emotional investment, long after they have given up hope. There is no clear-cut boundary between these two phases; Resolution begins to emerge in late Immersion, while Immersion issues may linger well into the Resolution phase.

Couples who have been able to remain connected while struggling with infertility will have an easier time dealing with Resolution than those couples who have not. When the latter group ends infertility treatment, they may find little to hold them together. The knowledge that a couple will not have a genetically related child represents the end of a dream and the beginning of Resolution—coming to terms with this loss.

11

⟡

COUPLE ISSUES IN THE RESOLUTION PHASE

"We got deeper and deeper into treatments. It took a
long time to realize how much time went by, how much
we lost touch with almost everything else. . . . We knew
we had to stop . . . we knew it was time. . . . I can't say
we're happy now, but in a way it's a relief to know we
tried everything. It's time to end."

CHARACTERISTICS OF RESOLUTION

In organizing an infertility self-help group with the mission of assisting
couples to move through and beyond the infertile experience, Barbara
Eck-Menning chose a particularly apt name: RESOLVE. This word
derives from Latin and the Middle English word *resolvere,* which means
to "unfasten," "loosen," or "release." Infertility can take hold of one's
identity; one's day-to-day life; one's emotions, thoughts, and relationships; and even one's bank account. Therefore, the process of disengage-
ment takes time.

The Resolution phase encompasses three overlapping tasks:

- *Ending medical treatment*—the decision to end all medical interventions.
- *Mourning*—the task of dealing with the reality of not having a
  genetically related child together and grieving the associated
  losses.

- *Refocusing*—the process of moving past the infertility experience by choosing either adoption or a life without children.

Couples may not accomplish these tasks in a linear progression: for example, a couple may be mourning their losses while still desperately continuing medical treatment in a last-ditch attempt at pregnancy. Or, having taken what they intended to be a short break or "sabbatical" from treatment, the partners may find themselves reengaging in their careers and social activities to the extent that they are reluctant to reinvest in medical treatments.

In general, couples come to a point at which they feel the loss more deeply, grieve, and then start to move away from the medical treatments:

> "Although we knew this was nuts—trying each time knowing we would probably lose—we kept doing it because we weren't ready to give up. But now we are. The decision was hard, and it still hurts a lot. But we've done our crying and screaming and being depressed. . . . We're tired—it's time to move on. We called the clinic today to say, 'Thanks, but no thanks.' "

Although sadness about the losses will return from time to time during the Legacy phase, and the feelings never fully disappear, couples who successfully grieve may have an easier time moving forward with their lives. Many of those who are unable to reach such a resolution continue to have regrets of what could have been.

The ordeal of infertility has four possible outcomes: Couples will emerge with either (1) a genetically related child, (2) a donor-conceived child, (3) an adopted child, or (4) no child. Those who have achieved a pregnancy through infertility treatments using their own gametes will spend a relatively brief time in Resolution, although there may be emotional and relational reverberations for years to come. Couples who have used donor gametes often begin to resolve their loss of a genetically related child in late Immersion, although they may have residual feelings of loss that need to be acknowledged in order to move forward. The crucial choice for those who have not achieved pregnancy during Immersion is deciding whether they will adopt or have a life without children.

ENDING MEDICAL TREATMENT

> "After months of preparations, the shots, the decision making, the disagreements, I couldn't go on. That is when I thought, 'I can't do this anymore. I'm finished.' "

Couples so caught up in getting pregnant may make treatment decisions in a perfunctory manner. In Immersion, couples may proceed almost automatically from one protocol to another, moving upward on the medical treatment ladder or repeating the same protocol over and over. Some couples continue with medical interventions until they have depleted their financial resources or treatment options. Howard and Lorraine, for example, came for couple therapy after 13 failed medical interventions; they were not only close to bankruptcy, but their marriage was headed toward a divorce.

However, many couples reach a point at which they feel so defeated by medical failures that they no longer have the emotional energy to rally for yet another treatment. Exhausted and unable to concentrate on any other part of life, they realize that their chances of achieving a pregnancy are slim at best. The following are some of the signs that couples are approaching the decision to stop medical treatment:

- Conscientious patients often become noncompliant, forgetting to take their medication or missing medical appointments: "I'm very tired of this cycle. I've been screwing up my own shots and hurting myself at night. I just feel very worn out."
- Although doctors' appointments may previously have been experienced as necessary ordeals, couples now respond to their physicians and the clinical procedures with anger and resentment.
- The partners have become increasingly conflicted or emotionally distant as they feel more and more discouraged with themselves and one another.
- Couples begin to take another look at alternatives to genetically related children; they begin to focus on parenting as opposed to getting pregnant, or they may weigh what life would be like without children.
- When there is secondary infertility, parents are increasingly distraught over how they may be neglecting their existing children.

Despite these signs of readiness, it may take couples time to decide to stop medical treatment, and some never completely give up hope of a pregnancy. One factor that allows couples to end treatment is the likelihood that they will not conceive. It is easier to accept the losses of infertility and move ahead if there has been a definitive diagnosis or if the couple believes that they have tried all possible treatments.

Endless Treatment

In the past, infertility treatments had an inevitable end point; with the advent of the new reproductive technologies, treatments can extend indefinitely. One reason that couples remain on the treatment path longer than seems reasonable is that they fear looking back with regrets over having rejected certain treatment or giving each procedure an insufficient number of trials. Governed by what might be termed *anticipatory regrets* (Sandelowski, 1993), these couples may be convinced that there is no use in trying, but they are unable to end medical treatment.

Some couples feel that neither adoption nor a life without children is acceptable. They continue the pursuit of treatment despite an accumulation of failures in order to protect themselves from accepting and dealing with the losses of infertility. When they eventually stop treatments and are forced to face these losses head on, grief reactions can be acute.

Treatment Failures

As treatment wears on and no baby is born, couples reach a point at which the repeated disappointments and losses that accompany either the onset of menstrual cycles or news of another failure become so chronic that the impact feels less traumatic. Existing hope becomes increasingly tempered by the memory of previous setbacks: "Who knows? It's a long shot, I don't really expect this [another procedure] will do anything," becomes the sentiment at the start of the cycle, and "Yes, we were disappointed, but not surprised" is likely to be the reaction when it ends in failure.

Research (Boivan et al., 1995) supports our clinical observations that it is the number of treatment failures, rather than the years spent in treatment or the couples' age, that predict personal distress and marital discord. Therefore, in the Resolution phase, couples' hopes of attaining pregnancy diminish as repeated failures mount, and they begin to consider ending further medical intervention.

Once the decision to abandon treatment is made, each person's reactions may differ. Although partners may agree that it is time to terminate medical treatment, some find living with the decision painful at first, while others are relieved; most experience both sets of feelings:

> An adoptive mother of two children looked back on the infertility stage of her life and said that ending treatment was "the hardest and the best decision we ever made. . . . It is impossible to describe the weight that was lifted off me; it wasn't until after it was over that I realized how heavy it was."

Impact on the Couple Relationship

As with other decisions made by couples, partners may not always be in agreement as to when they should stop treatment. Each partner seems to come to this decision in his or her own time, and each may require different sorts of "proof" before becoming ready to abandon treatment and refocus on other aspects of life. This particular negotiation—ending treatment and moving on to whatever comes next—is usually crucial for the couple; if either party feels it was arrived at prematurely, there are likely to be consequences in the future.

With some couples, each partner's position regarding continuing or ending treatment may be consistent over time. For example, one partner may be steadfast in insisting that any and all medical intervention should be undertaken to achieve a pregnancy, whereas the other partner opposes each procedure. In time, the partner advocating for treatment agrees to stop. For other couples, when it looks as though they are ready to end treatment, their positions may reverse.

The Couple and the Medical System

Unable to have a child, couples may experience a variety of emotions about their doctor, the clinic personnel, and the medical profession in general (Berg et al., 1991; Mahlstedt, 1985). Whereas some may feel angry and exploited by their medical providers, others, who have come to depend on these relationships, may find it difficult to let go of them (McDaniel et al., 1992). In addition, they may experience guilt at "letting down" the doctor who has tried so hard to help them. Occasionally, couples may find that their doctors encourage them to keep trying even when they have reached the their limit. Saying "No" can be difficult.

> Joan and Gerald decided to end treatment after several months of diagnostic tests followed by two IVF protocols that ended in second trimester miscarriages. Joan's physician thought she was abandoning treatment too soon because her chances of carrying a baby to term were quite good. But, in spite of his optimism, Joan felt that she could not subject herself to another loss, and she preferred to pursue adoption. Gerald would have liked to keep trying. However, seeing the toll it was taking on his wife and having no objection to adoption, he agreed that stopping treatment was the best choice for the couple.

For those couples who are able to achieve pregnancy using the expertise of infertility specialists, the shift to working with an obstetrician can be disappointing, because the involvement may be less intense and less personal than with an infertility specialist. Although they are relieved to give up infertility interventions, they may miss the special relationship they had with the clinic: "It's nothing like the loss [of a child] we were facing, but it's still a loss."

Sabbaticals

As the months or years devoted to becoming pregnant go by, some couples put medical treatment on hold without having specific plans about what they will do next. Made weary by sadness, distress, failure, and strained financial resources, their hope and enthusiasm about a medical solution peters out. Sometimes the decision to take a treatment "sabbatical" is deliberate, whereas other couples gradually drift away from the medical arena. While taking sabbaticals from treatment, couples may use their energy, previously devoted to the infertility treatments, to reconnect with friends and family members from whom they had become distant, and to reengage in their careers and interests. These couples may later return to infertility treatments if a strong desire for a child persists. Other couples decide not to return to the medical arena. Enjoying their renewed social and career activities, they may recognize the enormous emotional toll infertility treatments had taken on their lives. They begin to consider the other options: adoption or life without children.

Revisiting the Possibility of Medical Solutions: New Technology, Reawakened Hopes

Ending treatment is not always a final decision. The desire for a pregnancy may be reawakened after learning of a new reproductive procedure. For example, ICSI, a relatively recent ART procedure, overcomes the problem of poor quality sperm and thereby enables couples with male factor infertility to revisit the possibility of having a jointly conceived child. As medicine advances, and new reproductive technologies continue to push the fertility envelope, many more couples will be faced with the possibility of reopening the door to medical interventions. Some couples, feeling they have been granted an unexpected opportunity, choose to return to infertility specialists and pursue new protocols. They may again experience the same sequence of phases (albeit in an abbreviated form) that were part of their earlier involvement with infertility treatment. However, the second encounter with the medical world is often very different. The couples' expectations may be lower, and they may devote less time and energy to infertility treatments.

There will certainly be couples who are unwilling to reimmerse themselves in the distress and disappointment of trying to become pregnant. Nevertheless, they may still harbor the dream of having a genetically related child and have to revisit their decision over and over again.

"For the first 6 months after adopting our baby, I felt elated and that fate must have made me infertile so I could become a mother to this amazing child. But as time passed, I was surprised to find myself looking at pregnant women with the same old feelings of envy. But I still wasn't interested in returning to infertility treatments."

MOURNING

"We've tried everything. . . . This is taking too much out of us. It's time to move on. I think there's going to be a lot of sadness now."

Very few couples emerge from the infertility ordeal completely unscathed. Most continue to feel the pain of this experience. Moving on with one's life is facilitated by facing one's losses, mourning them, and making room for the sadness whenever it recurs. Couples who have successfully resolved their losses are still likely to feel sad from time to time and may experience the occasional pang of regret, no matter how much they enjoy their current lives. No matter what the outcome, feelings of grief, defectiveness, and shame may crop up unexpectedly. It is important to remember that having a child is not a "cure" for the emotional pain of infertility. Even those who have a fully genetically related child may still suffer from lingering feelings of defect and inadequacy. Likewise, and perhaps to a greater degree, couples with donor-conceived or adopted children may still harbor painful emotions about their ordeal, despite the happiness they may derive from parenthood.

Loss

During the Resolution phase, losses that have been experienced earlier now carry a sense of finality that can be devastating. Some of the earlier losses that are now faced more fully include the following:

- Loss of a jointly conceived, genetically related child.
- Loss of the childbearing stage in the life cycle.
- Loss of feeling a part of a child-centered community (and the resulting sense of being an outsider).
- Loss of the genetic continuity that links the past and future.
- Loss of control: Many experience their ultimate childlessness as a profound indication that the control they felt they had over their lives was merely an illusion.

Couples who are moving toward the choice of a life without children often feel deep sadness about the loss of a shared parenting experience, and may be concerned about what *will* hold them together. Grief can also be triggered by the reactions of others, such as when adoptive parents hear comments like, "I didn't notice you were pregnant," or "Who does the child look like?" Later, sadness may emerge when the parents prepare to tell the child about his or her adoption or donor origins. Overall, although brief episodes of grief can be expected to linger, couples who are able to acknowledge the sadness and comfort each other during Resolution are likely to continue this process into the future.

Adjusting to Pregnancy

Couples who achieve a pregnancy after years of infertility treatments may be more cautious as they enter into a pregnancy. Repeated failures have conditioned them to expect disappointment and can interfere with their bonding with the developing embryo. Sometimes difficulties in bonding may persist even after the baby is born:

> Erica was devastated when her first child was stillborn. With her second pregnancy, she could not muster much enthusiasm. Although the baby was born healthy, Erica still could not fully bond with the infant as she was worried about SIDS (sudden infant death syndrome). It was only after 3 months, when the danger of crib death was past, that she was able to connect with her baby.

The "Two-Track" Approach

Typically, adoption procedures are lengthy. Couples, especially those who realize that their childbearing years will soon be over, may look into adoption while they are still actively involved in fertility treatments, thus simultaneously pursuing two tracks to parenthood. These couples may believe that they will be able to make the necessary emotional adjustment to adoption. The focus on having a baby is so intense that many do not consider that there may be consequences to adopting while remaining totally invested in having "their own child." Couples may feel pressured because many agencies have age limits for adopting parents. In addition, birth parents are increasingly more involved in selecting their baby's new parent(s), so that "older couples" (often this means couples over 40) may be ruled out.

> Nat and Sarah tried to cover both bases, contacting an adoption agency while still actively engaged in the medical arena. Because they were unaware of the agency's concerns about pursuing both avenues simultaneously, they were candid about their ongoing

infertility treatments. In exploring their feelings about not having a genetically related child, the agency social worker made the assessment that they were not ready for adoption. Sarah was shocked and angry to learn that their application had been put on hold until their infertility treatments were completed. Nat, who had been less immersed in the treatment process and was more able to see the agency's perspective, thought the decision made sense.

Months later, during a recess in hormone injections, Sarah too realized that an adoption would indeed have been ill timed. One wonders what might have happened to the couple, and their adopted child, had they pursued a private adoption where emotional readiness for adoptive parenthood is not explored.

Differing points of view exist in the adoption field on the significance of resolving infertility and discontinuing infertility treatments prior to embarking on an adoption. Most adoption professionals believe that before moving into adoption, couples need to accept the probability that they will not give birth to a baby that is genetically related to them both. A few believe that a "two-track" system is an individual decision that does not necessarily affect the adoption outcome.

Clearly, emotional readiness for adoption is not a discreet event. Although many adopting parents continue to hold out some hope for that "miracle child," before they move into an adoption it is important for that hope to have faded significantly. As couples grieve, they become more able to face the prospect of having a family formed in a different way. Their focus shifts from "having a baby" to "becoming parents."

Initially, adoption can feel like a safety net for people whose hope of becoming biological parents is waning. Compared to the infertility treatments, these people believe that adoption is "a sure thing." However, many learn that the adoption process can be another roller coaster ride akin to infertility treatments.

REFOCUSING

"The battle with infertility has helped us get more solid and helped me believe in us more. I used to think our marriage wasn't going to last. But now I think it's the best thing since sliced bread."

As couples stop medical treatment and deal with their losses, they begin to focus on their lives, which had been placed on hold. Friends and family have often been pushed into the background, and career decisions deferred. In cases of secondary infertility, the needs of an existing child may have been ignored during the ordeal with infertility.

As couples begin to see an end approaching, refocusing can be marked by a sense of relief and an increase in energy. If couples do not have a child, there is often a bittersweet quality to this time as they acknowledge that things did not turn out as they had wished but that their lives can be full and meaningful just the same. The sadness, guilt, blame, and shame of previous phases begin to recede, and couples reach a more neutral emotional state. The task of refocusing, therefore, is one of making choices about how to live after infertility, and, for couples who did not have a child, the crucial choice will be between adoption and a childfree life. If they choose adoption, they accept that "We are not going to have child" and embrace the thought that "We can still be parents." In choosing a life without children, the idea is "We are not going to be parents, but we still have a life."

Impact on the Couple Relationship

The Resolution phase often marks a major turning point in a couple's relationship, particularly if they have not been able to have a child. Parents of a jointly conceived child often need to make adjustments when a child arrives regardless of whether or not they have experienced infertility, and those who conceive using donor gametes must grapple with the relational complexities involved. However, couples who are not able to give birth to a child and decide against adoption may be faced with the task of reexamining their entire relationship, especially if it was predicated on having a baby. In confronting the task of refocusing, they may need to take a hard look at the premises and expectations on which their relationship is based. Couples considering adoption also face important considerations.

Choosing Adoption

In Immersion, many couples refuse to consider adoption because it interferes with their ability to focus wholeheartedly on the medical treatment. Others decide against it because it is too emotionally complicated. However, in the Resolution phase, they may revisit the issue and make a different choice.

> George and Sally were "dead set against an adoption" after 2½ years of infertility treatments, and they could barely tolerate the therapist's questions about adoption. After another 2 years and a series of treatment failures, Sally hesitantly raised the topic of adoption only to find that George, too, had been wondering about revisiting the option. During their next session, they spoke about their

fears and prejudices concerning an adopted child, as well as the desire each had to be a parent. "I would have never thought we could even think about the possibility," said George, on the eve of flying to South America to take their adopted son home. "But we're not the people we were when we started this process," added Sally.

When couples near the end of the line in medical treatments, after the repeated failures, financial sacrifices, and a mounting sense of hopelessness, their thoughts begin shifting from "I want to have a baby" to "I want to be a parent." This shift can feel liberating. They begin to consider what is most essential and what they are willing to sacrifice. Aside from revisiting their goal of having a genetically related child, pregnancy, childbirth, and breastfeeding begin to seem less significant than the lifelong involvement with a child. Couples may focus on the "nurture" aspect as an important factor in the creation of a child's personality. Although in the past they may have registered only negative stories about adoption, they become increasingly attentive to stories about other couples' positive experiences.

For other couples, genetic legacies may be more important than parenting. They may feel that if the child cannot be of their genes, they are unwilling to undergo the trials of parenting. They may bolster their choice with negative reports about others' adoption experiences and decide that adoption is a poor choice for them.

Greg's older brother adopted a child whom the family considered the proverbial "bad seed." When family members learned that Greg and his wife, Christine, were experiencing infertility, they were relentless in pointing out the perils of adoption. Greg had many of his own negative associations to adoption and refused to consider it. Christine, although willing to consider adoption, felt impelled to abandon it: "I guess I'll have to make my peace with childlessness," she said. "It's not worth giving up my marriage."

In contrast, Daphne and Bill were devastated when they realized that they could never have a genetically related child. Although adoption was not their first choice, over time they came to see it as a "terrific option." Once they adopted, they could not imagine loving any child more.

Unfortunately, some couples adopt without confronting their sadness over their losses, often in order to avoid confronting the pain. As a consequence, their ability to accept the adopted child may be compromised as he or she represents their disappointment. Adoptive parents who have not come to terms with infertility—at least to some extent—can find it difficult to accept the birth parents as having significance to their child. Unfortunately, when children pick up their adoptive parents' discomfort with the birth parents, these children are likely to personalize such negative feelings and feel bad about themselves and the way in which their family was formed. Because infertility is the typical prelude to adoption, it is important to underscore how significant the Resolution phase is, not only for the couples, but for the adopted children as well.

Choosing Life without Children

Research has shown a significant number of couples report that marital satisfaction decreases after the birth of the first child and continues to decrease through the end of the child's third year (Belsky & Rovine, 1990). Couples without children can retain the spontaneity and freedom that parenthood curtails (Carter & Carter, 1989). When couples are unable to have children, some choose to live without them in spite of society's judgment that *not* having children is selfish and unnatural. When couples make this life choice, they often find it satisfying. However, such couples may feel guilty about reporting that their lives are going well: "When my cousins look at me and say how sorry they are that Josh and I can't have a baby, I feel like a fraud because secretly inside I'm thinking, 'I'm so glad I don't have to deal with kids.' I don't think I was meant to be a mother. I really don't miss it. What I mostly feel is relief."

There are many reasons why people consider a life without children. Some individuals may be so haunted by problematic family legacies and the fear of perpetuating them that they may go through the motions of becoming pregnant while feeling quite ambivalent about becoming parents. Couples with no problematic family legacies may simply choose not to have children. Couples who marry later in life, with the understanding that their chances of having a child are diminished, may be able to accept their infertility more easily than couples with higher expectations.

For couples who, out of choice or ambivalence, delay childbearing beyond their peak fertile years, the diagnosis of infertility can elicit complicated emotional responses. Although infertility can liberate them from the onus of deliberately choosing not to have children, the partners may still feel some shame at avoiding childbearing when it is so highly prized by the rest of society. These couples may linger in a limbo of half-hearted attempts to become pregnant before they move on with their lives.

Secrecy and Protection

As partners contemplate their future after infertility treatments have failed, they may have lingering feelings of blame, anger, and guilt. People often assume, incorrectly, that moving on means no longer feeling ambivalent or distressed. They might avoid talking about how much pain they still feel because they are unaware that resentments, lack of sexual desire, self-recriminations, and sadness are common.

Couples are likely to feel some apprehension about the future, whether it be life with an adopted child or no children. Partners worry that they will be disappointed with the child they adopt, or that they will have difficulty loving a child not born to them, but they may keep their concerns about adoption to themselves. Other couples harbor secret doubts about a life without children. Each partner may have unpleasant fantasies of the future, imagining he or she will be facing a void, or worrying about not being able to depend on children to care for them in their old age. Partners may ask themselves such questions as "Is my career going to be enough to sustain me? What are we going to talk about? What are we going to do together?" Partners can find it difficult to discuss these concerns with one another, out of protection of themselves, their partner, and the relationship, or out of concern that raising these feelings will be interpreted as doubting the decision not to have children.

Gender Differences

Parenting can be more central to the definition of womanhood than it is to manhood. Standing at the midway point in life and assessing their accomplishments, men tend to look more toward their careers for evidence of success, whereas women tend to define themselves and their contribution to posterity in terms of motherhood (Greil, 1991; Sandelowski, 1993).

> In their 50s, Andrea and her sister Debbie took stock. Debbie had three children, one in graduate school and the other two in college. Her career as a receptionist was minimally satisfying, undertaken mostly as a financial necessity for the family. Andrea, unable to have children, was a successful editor who found her career fulfilling. Yet Andrea had a profound ache and sense of "incompleteness" because she had never had children, whereas Debbie, though she regretted never pursuing "a real career," felt fulfilled. Andrea's husband, Peter, had a rewarding career and did not feel that something was lacking in his life: "Children would have been a great addition, but more like an extra—not central to how I see myself."

Reorientation to a life without children can be more complicated for women than for their partners. Most women assume they will be mothers and consequently leave a space in their lives for children. They, more than men, are likely to have made career decisions with this in mind choosing either to defer parenting, to sacrifice career advancements, or to relinquish a career altogether in favor of parenting. These women may find it particularly painful to abandon medical treatment, as their distress may not only be related to the loss of the child, but to the loss of motherhood. If they have not given this possibility much thought, it may be difficult and painful to envision their future lives.

Sexual Relationship

As described earlier, a couple's sex life is often adversely affected by the encounter with infertility. In this phase, as partners refocus their attentions on their lives, sexual problems that developed earlier may come into the foreground as coping with the infertility recedes.

The Couple with the Support System

As couples refocus on themselves, they resume their prior lives and reengage in relationships with friends and family members. Although the painful isolation of the earlier phases is not missed, some couples may have established patterns of separateness from their families of origin that they are reluctant to give up. If couples were overly enmeshed with their families of origin or families were intrusive in their affairs, they may enjoy the distance and privacy they took or were given because of the infertility. But if they have a child, whether through pregnancy or adoption, the families generally want to be more involved in the threesome's life.

> Danielle's mother-in-law wanted to redecorate the child's room, whereas Danielle preferred to wait until she and her husband, Ron, could do it together. Whereas before she would have welcomed her mother-in-law's offer, infertility had made the couple a team, and she preferred planning for the baby with her husband.

When the reengagement of a family member is welcomed and appreciated, couples may wish to continue their independent position at the same time as they step closer to their families. They may need to set clearer boundaries than they had in the past.

Reentering the family circle after deciding not to have children can present challenges. Couples must be prepared for what may well be a life-long position in which others feel free to ask personally intrusive questions and express their opinions—rarely positive—about the couple's life choice.

SECONDARY INFERTILITY

After months, perhaps years, spent in infertility treatment, many couples struggling with secondary infertility come to feel more and more uncomfortable with the fact that their focus on having another child is taking so much energy away from the child they do have. This often becomes the impetus to end medical treatment; they no longer wish to miss out on the precious moments of the existing child's youth:

> "I feel like I lost a year of my life with my daughter. I don't know what happened. . . . God, it went by so fast. I'm afraid in wanting to expand my family, I'm not going to really be with the family we have now."

Although such couples may mourn the loss of their ideal family—including size of family, sex of children, and a desired spacing between children—the child they have often becomes that much more valuable to them, particularly if they decide against either donor or adoption procedures.

Some couples are very committed to having a larger family and so may consider adoption. If they make that choice, they often face considerable social censure. Many people believe that the parents are looking for trouble, that they will love their genetically related child more and that the relationship between the siblings will be compromised. Indeed, some parents may start out with the assumption that the adopted child will have so much to deal with in life, they want to protect the child from additional adversity. In these situations, parents may overcompensate by treating the adopted child differently. For example, they may avoid talking about the excitement of the first child's birth, hoping to spare the adopted child any feelings of envy. They do not realize that they can tell joyful stories about how each child entered the family. Although it requires thoughtful planning and emotional awareness to overcome the complex relationships in such family constellations, these kinds of considerations are more likely to be faced by couples who not only are certain that they want more than one child, but are comfortable with the choice they have made.

12

⮂

THERAPEUTIC APPROACH
IN THE RESOLUTION PHASE

> Infertility symbolizes the loss of the future. It is not
> possible to move on with life until the future has been
> reorganized in a person's mind and given new meaning.
> On the broadest level, resolution necessitates finding
> what was lost: the meaning of life. The life story must
> be constructed to fit a different set of circumstances than
> those originally anticipated. To do this entails the
> preparation of a place in the life story for an altered set
> of hopes and dreams. In this reorganization process, new
> room is created—freed up for new and different kinds of
> hopes and ideas to be entertained.
> —BECKER (1990, P. 236)

PRESENTING PROBLEM

Couples who have been in therapy during Immersion begin moving
toward the Resolution phase as repeated failures and the accompanying
distress mount. As they lean more toward the idea of ending medical
treatment, the clinician can be alert to cues that they are moving into
Resolution. Some of the signs are increased resentment of or noncompli-
ance with medical treatments, emotional exhaustion, and, most significantly, a focus less on pregnancy and more on the wish to parent. Some
may also think more seriously about the possibility of choosing a life
without children.

Adoption is a major life choice that is likely to be made in Resolution. Couples may come to therapy with conflicts about adoption including (1) being out of synch with each other regarding readiness to adopt (e.g., one partner may be comfortable moving forward while the other wants to continue medical treatment, or one partner is open to the adoption process while the other is fiercely opposed) or (2) having issues to work through before they are ready to take this step, primarily grieving the loss of not having a genetically related child.

In this phase, one of the clinician's primary tasks is to help couples talk about and resolve their losses so they are comfortable with whichever choice they make: adoption or life without children. Part of this process may include helping the couple grieve their losses through mourning rituals. As couples are no longer focused on getting pregnant, partners take stock of their lives, including their relationship. It may be that during Resolution relational patterns that were tolerated during Immersion are no longer acceptable. If these are not addressed, the couple may move into the future burdened by pain and resentment. For some, the healing process seems too difficult to tackle, especially after the ordeal of infertility. They may lean toward dissolving the relationship.

> Sean and Tina came for therapy on the verge of separation. They were in the Resolution phase, having spent 4 years in Immersion with multiple, unexplained miscarriages. Sean was having an affair and spoke openly about his wish to have his own genetically related child with his lover. The therapist worked briefly with the couple to help them with the mourning process, but Sean abruptly left treatment to move in with his lover. Subsequently, he left the second relationship when they were unsuccessful in conceiving, and he wanted to reunite with Tina. She, having remained in therapy, had grieved her inability to have a child, and was uninterested in resuming the marriage.

THE THERAPIST'S ROLE

During Resolution, some partners may give the appearance of being in agreement about their decisions, whether they are choosing to end medical treatment, adopt, or live without children. Clinicians may, therefore, give little thought to challenging what appears to be a mutual choice. It is important for the clinician to determine whether the couple has fully discussed the issue, or if either partner still has doubts. The clinician must probe to be sure that the partners have chosen this track because they both feel it would be best, rather than because they cannot tolerate any more fighting and tension in the relationship.

Because the choices made during Resolution have long-term significance, in this phase it is important for the therapist to separate his or her biases from the couple's choices. For example, a therapist who has a genetically related child may think a couple's choice to adopt or to proceed without children has been too hastily made and that they ought to try more medical procedures. On the other hand, a therapist who has adopted may think the couple should adopt rather than abandon parenting all together. Once again, we assume that by identifying his or her own beliefs, a therapist is less likely to impose them on the couple.

LOCATE THE COUPLE ON THE TRAJECTORY

Resolution is not always an easy phase to identify: It has three overlapping subphases—ending medical treatment, mourning, and refocusing—and it is a phase that may last a long time. When couples have been in Immersion, the first signs that they are moving towards Resolution may be that they have more conversations about the non-baby-related aspects of their lives. They may talk more about their careers, thoughts of moving, and growing interests in new activities. Because they no longer face the ticking clock of biology, they have the luxury of taking their time to make these significant decisions.

WORKING WITH THE COUPLE: TREATMENT ISSUES, TECHNIQUES, AND STRATEGIES

As couples consider ending medical treatment and come to terms with their losses, they often feel as if they are reawakening from a dream. Realizing how infertility has taken over their lives, they begin to imagine moving out of the limbo of infertility and back into "regular" life. At the same time, couples begin to express their distress over the state of their emotional and social lives.

Restructuring the Relationship

Couples in Resolution who opt for a life without children must make a major shift in the way they had envisioned their relationship (Peoples & Ferguson, 1998). During Immersion, the focus on parenthood overshadowed many other aspects of the couple's life. Therefore, when medical treatment ends, the couple is left to consider "What now? Who are we now? What will we be in the future if there is no child?" Because the dyad tends to be the most unstable relationship configuration, children can stabilize couples in a variety of ways over the course of a marriage:

- The responsibilities of parenting organize and connect partners.
- Because children continue to develop and change, there are a variety of challenges, joys, and difficulties to share.
- In times of conflict, couples are less inclined to separate and divorce because they are concerned about the child's well-being and their own loss in not being in their child's daily life.

The prospect of life together without this unifying factor can raise uncomfortable thoughts and feelings. The success of Resolution may depend on how well couples have weathered the infertility process itself. If couples have not been able to work together as a couple or to get professional help, there are likely to be lingering resentments about decisions and feelings that were misunderstood or disqualified. This build-up of pain and resentment is likely to hamper the refocusing process. Without a child, these unresolved feelings may lead couples to seek out affairs or drift apart.

Partners who remain without children may engage in outside interests to stabilize the relationship and give them a common purpose There are a variety of ways of redefining the relationship and refocusing the couples' energy, for example, a couple may renovate an old house, start a new business, or get a pet. The search for new meaning and purpose can be a rewarding one and can strengthen and deepen the couple's relationship. For these couples, this enhanced awareness provides great satisfaction.

Many couples intuitively figure out how to redefine or restructure the marriage without the assistance of a therapist. The process gradually evolves with the realization that there will not be a child. Restructuring often begins earlier in the infertility experience as couples think about why they want to parent and have children; infertility often leads people to ask themselves existential questions and to ponder the meaning of their lives. So, as the possibility of life without children looms, they may already have begun to think about alternatives. However, in instances where one partner may wish to put more energy into the relationship, whereas the other may prefer to focus on work, new areas of conflict may arise.

Couples who have a shared focus begin to consider options that would have been ruled out had they had children. When couples appear to be struggling with this major life transition, the clinician might suggest that they find other couples in a similar position, try out different activities, or simply contemplate their choices.

When Nicki and Roger decided not to adopt, Nicki became more involved in her work as a freelance set designer. She became more assertive in making work contacts and began to take jobs out of town—something she had avoided during her ordeal with infertility. Therapy focused on how she and Roger might recapture the enjoyment of each other's company that had existed before the infertility was diagnosed.

EXPLORE COUPLES' BELIEF SYSTEMS

The Choice between Adoption and Life without Children: The Importance of Parenting

The Resolution process forces couples to consider the value they place on having a child. When it seems clear there will be no genetically related child, couples need to weigh the importance of parenting itself, even in the absence of a genetic connection with their child. Couples who have not yet considered adoption, or who set it aside as they tried to have a child, may begin to consider it at this time. As couples weigh the options of adoption or life without children, the therapist can again ask relevant questions about parenting and children.

Choosing Adoption

When faced with adoption as the one remaining method of becoming parents, some couples hastily embrace this option (to make up for all the time lost during infertility treatments) without adequately exploring whether they are comfortable with adoption and if it is a good choice for them.

Prospective adoptive parents are faced with many myths and misconceptions about adoption:

- A good adoptive family makes up for the loss of the birth family.
- If the adoptive parents are good parents and love the child enough, he or she will not want to search for the birth parents.
- Adopting internationally, with no possibility of a reunion, will lessen the significance of the birth parents, and the child will think about them less.
- Adoption is a cure for infertility.
- Once parents adopt a child, the losses of infertility will disappear.

People naively believe that if they can love an adopted child as they would their genetically related child, they are ready to adopt. Many couples approach adoption with the assumption that parenting an adopted child requires nothing more or less than parenting a child born to them, except for having to explain the adoption. This rationale may be intended to express comfort with adoption, but instead it conveys ignorance regarding the complexities and unique challenges adoption raises.

In spite of the individual nature of each family's adoption, there are universal adoption themes that impact on all members of the adoption circle, birth parents, adoptees, and adoptive parents; primarily *loss* and *loyalty* for everyone, and the *search for self*, which impacts most on adoptees, who often face a life-long quest to understand what it means to be adopted. Clinicians working with couples considering adoption need to be aware of these themes, of how they play out, and how to prepare couples to deal with them.

The therapist needs to remind couples that adoptive parenting is different from parenting genetically related children in that adoption is predicated on loss. Adoptive parents are frequently reminded that their child was not born to them. Reminders come from the comments of strangers who ask, "Where did she get that beautiful red hair?", from a school's questions about the child's prenatal environment, or the child saying, "You can't tell me what to do. You're not my real mother/father!"

The clinician should also point out that it will be the adoptive parents' task to help their child understand what it means to be adopted, and that this awareness is often accompanied by feelings of hurt and rejection. Adjustment to adoption is a life-long process. As the children grow and develop, and their intellectual and cognitive capacities to understand mature and deepen, adoptive parents must be responsive to their continued need to understand this complex process. Good adoptive parenting requires that parents understand and accept the significance of the birth family to their child (and to them) and expand their definition of family to include the birth family, regardless of whether the child will ever meet them.

In working with couples considering or in the process of adopting, the clinician can help them explore their motivation to adopt, understand the meaning adoption has for them, and examine the challenges of adoption and their willingness to handle these challenges. The following situations are examples of problematic premises that should alert clinicians to ambivalence, unresolved infertility, or a lack of readiness to adopt on the part of partners or the couple.

Denial of Loss

Although there are some people who do not feel any regret in connection with their infertility, for most, as stated earlier, the ordeal involves losses that must be acknowledged and grieved. The therapist needs to question the motives of couples who apply to adopt without seeking medical consultation for their infertility, couples who insist that it makes no difference whether they parent a child who is born to them or adopted, and couples who prefer to adopt.

If couples succeed in adopting a child without acknowledging, mourning, and to some extent resolving the losses of their infertility, the child may be burdened by the parents' implicit prohibition against the child acknowledging any of his or her own feelings of sadness and loss. The clinician can make the couple aware that by denying any differences between adopting and having a genetically related child, adoptive parents, in a sense, eradicate the child's connection to the birth parents and seemingly render it irrelevant. This, in turn, denies the child a chance to grieve, to work through his or her feelings of being different, and to heal the losses of adoption.

Adopting for Altruistic Reasons

Occasionally, families who already have children may adopt a special needs child in order to repay society for their own good fortune. However, most infertile couples adopt in order to become parents, in other words, for the same reasons that motivate fertile couples. When couples who have experienced infertility emphasize humanitarian motives over self-centered ones when considering adoption, clinicians need to be alert to the possibility that they are avoiding the losses of infertility and replacing them with charitable motives. It is as if the parents are saying, "If we felt sad about not having a genetically related child, we wouldn't be able to love you." This is the kind of either/or thinking that permeated the adoption field in the 1950s, that is, either you belong to your birth family or you belong to your adopted family. Therefore, this situation can cue the therapist to explore issues of loss further.

Denying the Existence or Significance of the Birth Parents

Adoptions today, compared to even a few years ago, involve much more openness between the birth parents and adoptive parents and, in open adoption, between the birth parents and the child. This change reflects a shift away from the closed adoption system of the past, which, unfortunately, was built on secrecy and engendered feelings of shame. Clinicians need to be aware of these shifts in order to provide a context for prospective adoptive parents+ anxieties, preferences, and attitudes regarding birth parents.

It is natural for couples who are considering adoption initially to feel uneasy and threatened by the openness that accompanies many adoptions today. Usually, that uneasiness dissipates when it becomes clear that openness is considered to be in the best interests of adopted children and their families. But concern on the part of the clinician is appropriate in any of the following situations: when prospective adoptive parents continue (1) to be uncomfortable about the birth parents, (2) to hold negative and judgmental views about them, (3) to prefer not to meet or correspond with them, or (4) if international adoption is chosen in order to avoid involvement with the birth parents. Couples who cannot relinquish their initial concerns and hesitations regarding birth parents are not yet ready for adoptive parenting, and the therapist can help them to understand the challenges involved.

Hesitation, Ambivalence, and Self-Protection

Some couples may be quite comfortable with adoption, are open to birth parents, and have come to terms with the infertility. However, they have been through so many infertility- and adoption-related losses that they are not able to feel the joy and excitement of adoption until the child is in their arms.

It is crucial for clinicians to understand that resolution is a fluid process, not a finite state. People who have experienced infertility losses never fully forget, and they face reminders of what might have been, particularly at life-cycle junctures.

Emily was adopted at birth and maintained a close and warm relationship with her adoptive parents as an adult. When she married and became pregnant, she and her mother, Fran, felt that because Fran had never experienced pregnancy and childbirth she could not be a resource to Emily. As one way to remedy the situation, and avoid experiencing additional losses, Emily and her husband invited Fran to be Emily's childbirth coach and to be with them in the delivery room. In this way, Emily and her mother could share the experience.

Choosing Life without Children

Choosing a life without children can be a difficult decision, as it runs counter to conventional social expectations. It is often difficult to distinguish society's dictums from one's own desires, and couples may feel a certain embarrassment, even shame, about their decision. Men may feel more comfortable choosing to forego parenting than women, however women are increasingly able to reconceptualize their roles in life and society, and thereby achieve their identity and satisfaction from roles other than that of "mother" (Ireland, 1993).

If couples are leaning toward a life without children, the clinician will want to ascertain, as with adoption, that they are not rushing ahead and bypassing the process of mourning. Whereas the active involvement in the adoption process offers an easier escape from grief, couples without children may try to deny their grief by throwing themselves into their work or other activities. In their desperation to keep busy, they leave little time or energy for their relationships. Because the partners' recent experiences of intimacy were filled with pain and loss, they may become increasingly distant and isolated from each other.

Most couples who have encountered infertility seem to approach the decision of living without children after thoughtfully considering many of the implications. However, like the surprises that come with having children (e.g., parents are likely to be overwhelmed by the depth of love they have for a child or by how angry they can get with a child who defies them), many of the future ramifications of life without children are not anticipated. A couple that elects not to have children may be taken unawares by the feelings that surface years after the decision is made.

> Ellen, after making the decision not to have children, recounted the following story: "The other day I was visiting my friend, and we were both playing with her daughter. The little girl fell down and hurt herself. I tried to help her up, but she just cried, 'Mommy, Mommy.' What I will miss most is that there will never be anyone for whom I am the most important person in the world, who will come running to *me* when they are hurt."

Because there may be few models of others who have chosen life without children in the couple's circle of friends and family, the clinician can help couples think about their choice and the issues that might arise in the future.

In raising the following questions, our expressed intention is not to challenge couples' decisions, but to prepare them for the future they may face as the result of having chosen to take a nontraditional path:

- When you explore this together, what are the pros and cons of this decision?
- Who is more interested in a life without children?
- Do you think it will affect your relationship? In what way?
- How do each of you imagine your individual lives will be different than had you had children?

- What do you think your family will say?
- What do you think you might miss?
- What do you think you would value?

FACILITATE MOURNING

"In the concentration camps, the women would stop menstruating; there was a definite interruption of the reproductive cycle there, at least from the women's point of view. And so you had this sense that one side of you was being annihilated, that on one level of your life, everything that you assume is going to happen stops. Everything. Everything else in my life goes on, but on this very basic level, it's not going on. . . . We can have [donor-conceived or adopted] children, yes, and we can have a family. But that part of me, that one that wanted to continue all the history I know, it's ending in that one area" (Ackerman Institute for the Family's Infertility Project, 1995).

Mourning and the Couple

Couples typically imagine how it will be to create a child. This vision affects the way they see themselves, their partner, their relationship, and their expectations about how they will relate to family, friends, and the world at large. When couples are forced to abandon their mutually held idea of having a child, their grief is not only about the loss of the imagined child, but also about being denied the opportunity to create a child together. Although partners may grieve separately, they may not always grieve as a couple. Mourning together allows for the expression of each partner's sadness over his or her losses, and for mutual grieving for their losses as a couple.

While pregnant with a DI-conceived son, Mary said to her husband, Donald, "It's a loss for both of us, and it's a loss for you, and it's a loss for me. . . . I think that it really is a loss for me as an individual. . . . I know that your loss is profound and unthinkable, Donald . . . but I really . . . feel a profound sense of loss, too."

Partners who are uncomfortable sharing their grief, perhaps to spare the other, may find themselves growing more distant. Sometimes resentment builds when one or both feel their grief is misunderstood, or they feel constrained to stifle their sadness. When painful emotions such as sadness are suppressed, depression, hostility, and generalized disaffection may occur.

Sometimes one partner, usually the woman, may be so protective of the other that he or she will deliberately conceal grief. However, the protected partner is then prevented from rising to meet the psychological challenge of hearing his or her partner's pain, and learning how to give comfort and support. When one partner does all the grieving, the other partner is denied the opportunity to mourn (Burns, 1990).

As couples work through their grief, the therapist can suggest they design and participate in a more formal grieving ritual. For example, one couple wrote a letter to their unborn child and read it during the session; another had a Mass performed; a third planted a memorial tree. As discussed earlier, raising the possibility of a ritual often leads couples to create unique rituals of their own, which may draw on their particular religious or spiritual traditions.

> When it became clear that Nancy and Bernard were never going to have a genetically related child, the therapist raised the idea of a ritual to mourn this loss. They turned to their cultural traditions and sat Shiva (a Jewish mourning ritual in which friends and relatives spend time with the grieving family). Whereas formal Shiva lasts a week, the couple planned it for only one night. This represented a formal demarcation of the passing of their dream of genetic parenthood and the loss of the child that they had wanted. Relatives and friends found it extremely helpful because they had felt awkward about how to share their own grief and to offer their condolences to the couple. The public mourning—a ritual—validated the loss. Although they had begun adoption proceedings, the Shiva helped clear the way for them to move forward with greater peace of mind.

EXPLORE RELATIONSHIP
WITH SUPPORT SYSTEM

Adoption

When couples consider adoption, they are offered a great deal of unsolicited advice and caution from well-intentioned friends and relatives. Implicitly or explicitly, this advice may be either encouraging or discouraging based on the experiences and attitudes of advice givers. Insensitive and negative attitudes toward adoption may be troubling for the parents-to-be, as such attitudes can heighten the couple's own ambivalence and deprive them of needed support from others. The therapist can help the couple plan how they might want to set limits with respect to their conversations with unsupportive friends and relatives.

Adoption disclosure, as with donor disclosure, can raise worries and concerns in the most well-adjusted adoptive parents. They wonder, "Will my child feel rejected when he or she learns what adoption means? Will he or she feel I love him or her less because I didn't give birth to him or her?" In terms of disclosure, we agree with our colleague Evan Imber-Black's position that the child "owns" the secret and therefore is entitled to know the truth about his or her origins.

When couples are considering adoption, or have already adopted, it is important for the clinician to ask them when and how they plan to tell their child about adoption (see Chapter 14), whether or not they have discussed this issue, whether they agree about how to proceed, and if not, where they disagree. If couples are concerned about the consequences of others knowing of the adoption, the clinician needs to remind them that once their child knows, the information is out of their control. They can be a resource to their child in helping him or her deal with the reactions of others, but they ought not withhold the information in order to protect their child from possible negative consequences.

Life without Children

Reengagement with family can be difficult for couples who have chosen not to have children. Having already been out of step with the rest of the family during their struggle with infertility, it may be a shock to reenter the flow of life when their expectations and plans have changed so radically. Some couples who have deliberately chosen not to have children may find it relatively easy to tell their families about their decision and to limit any discussion about the validity of their choice. Others, however, may be so uncomfortable discussing their decision that they find their reengagement with families very difficult. Nonetheless, it seems reasonable to share some information. Anticipating that their families will have questions, the couple may wish to take the initiative, in order to avoid further questions and advice, and tell family and friends that they have stopped trying to have a baby. The therapist can ask the couple about how they plan to deal with the questions that will inevitably arise at this reentry phase. This is also a time to encourage partners to talk about their ideas with each other and find a common ground regarding what they wish to share with others.

Couples who have chosen a life without children may decide to take a more active role in the lives of their nieces, nephews, or godchildren. They may wish to invite children for visits and attend special events such as school plays or Little League games. Alternatively, these couples may fulfill their desire to nurture children in some other way such as volunteer work or becoming a Big Brother or Big Sister.

> Greg and Christine, having tried unsuccessfully to have children for 10 of their 15 years together, each found different ways of engaging their desire to "leave our mark on the future generation." Greg, a gifted musician, became active in a local children's choral society

and spent much of his free time in rehearsing the children and fund raising on their behalf. Christine preferred to pass along her "legacy of having lived in this world" by spending time with her nieces.

EXPLORE THE RELATIONSHIP WITH THE CHILD

Disclosure with Adoption

A primary task for clinicians in Resolution is to ensure that couples have sufficiently mourned their losses such that they feel relatively comfortable discussing their child's origins with him or her, on an ongoing basis (see Chapter 14 for a detailed discussion of disclosure). Without a successful Resolution phase, parents may see adoption as being an inferior way to create a family. Parents may then worry about disclosure, projecting their own ideas onto the child and fearing that the child will feel that adoption gives him or her an inferior status. On the other hand, if people really feel that adoption is a fine way to have children, they will be less worried about the child being distressed to learn about his or her adoption.

However, no matter how comfortable parents may be about the adoption, children still need to deal with their feelings of loss. Parents who have not addressed their own losses are less likely to initiate these discussions with their child. Either they bring up the topic of adoption once and never mention it again, assuming they have explained it fully and the child understands it, or they take a stance that adoption is better than having their own genetically related child, by saying, for example, that they would never have had a child this smart, talented, and so forth. In either case, children are denied access to the most important resource they have to help them grieve—their parents.

With secondary infertility it is important to tell the biological child(ren) about the impending adoption. The more these children are involved in the adoption process, the easier it will be for them to understand how it works and to help them be a part of the new child's arrival into the family.

EXPLORE THE RELATIONSHIP WITH THE MEDICAL SYSTEM

Ending Medical Treatment

Couples may continue in medical treatments when it seems decreasingly likely that further intervention will succeed. The following may contribute to staying on the treadmill of continued treatment:

- Difficulty in mourning the hoped-for genetically related child.
- Difficulty in giving up the romance of pregnancy and childbirth.
- Prejudice against adoption, and actual negative experiences with the adoptive process.
- The need to ensure status via genetic reproduction within a family or community.
- The physician's promises of success.
- Any profoundly personal belief system that requires bearing a child.

Therefore, it is useful for the therapist to explore what keeps the couple stuck in endless treatment and prevents them from moving on.

TERMINATION: ENDING COUPLE THERAPY

As couples accomplish the steps of Resolution, the clinician can begin to increase the intervals between sessions and to initiate telephone contacts rather than having face-to-face meetings. At the conclusion of therapy, a more formal, final session can be scheduled in which the therapist encourages the couple to talk about how they have handled the infertility, what adversity has taught them as individuals and as a couple, and how they might use their experience to cope with other problems in the future. We prefer to leave the door open for couples to return to therapy if the infertility should overwhelm them again, making it explicit that returning for a "tune-up" does not mean that they have failed in any way.

END OF RESOLUTION

As the Resolution phase comes to a close, many couples report improved functioning. For these couples, their connection to each other has grown stronger as they learned to operate as a team in order to overcome the ordeal of infertility. They often find that they can resolve conflict and communicate better. "We came out of this much stronger as a couple. Our relationship now seems better than most couples we know."

Some couples, however, leave Resolution with an abiding sense of sadness and regret that they may carry into Legacy. If they are unable to make peace with their circumstances, their grief may affect their relationship and their children (if any), including the ability to help their children cope with donor and adoption issues as they arise.

Just as when someone dies, one may still experience bouts of sadness yet be able to move ahead and fulfill other dreams. Couples who have mourned the losses of infertility will, ideally, find important things to embrace, despite their lingering pain. Recognizing that the yearning may never fade, couples move ahead with a common purpose, prepared for sadness and expecting joy.

> "The medical confirmation of infertility came as a tidal wave, a Tsunami. We were each smashed and separated by it. . . . Now, it comes at us like waves that seem to go on forever. But we know how to handle the waves now, to hang on to each other. We go with them and let them carry us a little, and then get back to where we were."

13

⊕

COUPLE ISSUES IN THE LEGACY PHASE

> "When I see pregnant women or hear a friend is pregnant, I cringe for a second. That old pang returns. I still long to be pregnant again, even though parenting is wearing me out. I don't know if that feeling ever goes away."

CHARACTERISTICS OF LEGACY

Legacy, the aftermath of infertility, is the phase in which couples have moved on to the next chapter in their lives and any long-term effects of infertility are seen. Many couples report that, no matter what the \eventual outcome vis-à-vis children, infertility is a watershed event. Life is never quite the same afterward. For some couples, the repercussions can be so powerful that they are still felt decades later.

Leslie and Richard, a couple in their mid-60s, came to therapy wanting to improve their relationship. Complaints included "poor communication" and "bad sex." In exploring their history, two traumatic events were revealed: infertility some 30 years ago and a recent incidence of colon cancer. The therapist was surprised to discover that the infertility loomed larger in their minds as a source of discord, distress, and conflict. In fact, Richard's recent cancer primarily stirred up feelings about not leaving a genetic heir.

Regardless of how well partners have dealt with infertility, many experience recurring sadness either at key points in the life cycle, or simply out of the blue when some memory is evoked. They become used to the waves of sadness: "There's my old friend. It will always be a part of me" (Menning, 1988, p. 122). It is also important to remember that a baby—even one born "naturally"—is rarely the antidote or cure for infertility; some remnant of the infertile identity usually remains.

The more problematic aspects of Legacy are present in couples who have not come to terms with infertility and continue to be angry at and victimized by the experience. Left unaddressed to fester in silence, these legacies can affect the couple's behavior in such ways as ongoing sexual problems, communication difficulties, and parenting insecurities. Vivian's view of the aftermath of infertility seems typical: "I realized . . . the infertility doesn't go away. This [their donor-conceived baby] is such a wonderful thing, and we're so happy, but . . . what happened to us and the fact of Larry's infertility, it's never going to go away."

Nevertheless, there are couples who experience infertility as an acute (but temporary) condition; once remedied by medical treatment, spontaneous pregnancy, or adoption, infertility no longer holds great significance, nor does the aftermath carry such emotional weight.

LOSS

Although the crisis and trauma of infertility fade as time passes, the sense of loss may linger for years. Whereas shared loss can create a profound bond, when partners are unable to share their grief, they may live for years feeling estranged. Couples without children, and the bonds created by coparenting, need to restructure their relationship in order to avoid exacerbating their feelings of disconnection.

Any of the losses of infertility—a normal conception and pregnancy, sharing the creation of a genetically related child, and genetic continuity along family lines—may revisit the couple at any time. For example, when a woman who was unable to have children hears that her best friend's daughter is pregnant, she may feel a flood of sadness that she will not have grandchildren or experience the intimacy of sharing pregnancy stories with her daughter. Even decades later, unexpected circumstances can trigger painful feelings.

Maura had an extreme reaction when her stepchildren's offspring called her "Grandma," and she angrily demanded that they stop using the word. The therapist wondered whether this signified an awakening of Maura's own grief and anger over her infertility. In exploring her reaction within the context of her infertility, Maura realized that by not allowing the children to call her Grandma, she was protecting herself against the pain of both her loss and her jealousy because the stepchildren were able to conceive.

IMPACT ON THE COUPLE RELATIONSHIP

Many couples find that because they are united in adversity, they feel closer and more connected to each other. Postinfertile couples often report that the crisis resulted in improved marital communication and higher levels of marital satisfaction (Greil, 1991), and many feel more positive about their marriage after parenthood (Burns, 1990). If they entered therapy to learn to cope with the ordeal of infertility, they may have explored issues that they might not otherwise have confronted, and therefore experienced growth both personally and as a couple.

> Throughout the early phases of infertility, Sarah and Nat's characteristic style was to cope with each setback or loss by either not talking about it or having a nasty fight. In therapy, they were able to talk more openly about the disappointments of infertility while offering and accepting each other's support. As a result, they were better able to handle other aspects of their lives and marriage that had given them problems in the past. They both felt the infertility had made their relationship much stronger. Nat said that the infertility was "like a grain of sand in an oyster; we now have a pearl."

Couples experiencing a major trauma such as infertility are likely to have gained more understanding and wisdom and consequently feel more prepared to face life's hardships. Many feel a deep sense of gratitude for what they have. While friends gripe over relatively trivial difficulties, couples who became parents after infertility may appreciate parenthood more deeply and weather the travails with a bit more equanimity.

For couples who have chosen to remain childfree, they have many options for refocusing their lives. They can take greater risks in terms of career knowing they are not responsible for the welfare of children. Additionally, because they do not have to think about their children's college tuition and future inheritance, they have more money to spend without the pressures to save.

Secrecy and Protection

If the pattern of protectively hiding one's innermost thoughts and feelings from the other takes hold and persists, potential problems in the relationship are likely to increase. Couples may hide their sadness (e.g., crying silently during the baby commercials), their resentment, and their sense of guilt. Each partner may even suspect what the other is thinking or feeling (e.g., at a family event, when both are thinking, "Our child would have been this age"), but they say nothing. Unable to express themselves during Legacy, communication gaps that developed during the acute phases of infertility may widen. Partners who sought to protect each other from guilt and resentment often continue the same patterns of silence and avoidance years after the immediate crisis of infertility has passed. Some may have turned to friends or individual therapists for solace and understanding during the ordeal, never resuming intimate communication with their partners. These rifts, whether angry or silent, can be hard to bridge.

Without some essential refocusing of their marriages, couples without children may find themselves, years later, less satisfied with their choices than they had hoped. They may feel an emptiness along with a sense that their relationships are not enough to sustain them. Each partner may have found different ways to replace the void, which have moved them in different directions. One partner may be wanting more connection and self-fulfillment within the relationship, while the other is content with less intimacy and more involvement in outer-directed activities. Partners may not talk about their remorse over the decisions that they have made.

Gender Differences

Life after infertility, like the phases that preceded it, may be different for each partner. Because women are likely to be the more distressed partners, their lives may change more and it may take longer for them to heal. Women may experience more social discomfort because their social lives tend to center around children, whereas men have other areas of connection. After retirement age, children and grandchildren become a major topic of discussion for many women, and those who struggled with infertility may find social gatherings painful reminders.

Sexual Relationship

During Immersion, couples often find that trying to get pregnant and sustain a passionate sexual relationship become mutually incompatible. In Legacy, when couples are asked about their sex lives, they often report problems. These sexual difficulties can be manageable or catastrophic for the couple, depending on the importance of sex in their relationship and the meaning they attach to its absence. For some couples, sex is such a fundamental way of achieving intimacy that its absence can have significant and negative consequences on the couple's relationship. As their enjoyment of sex diminishes, the ability to use physical intimacy as a means of achieving and reinforcing their emotional connection is severely compromised. If they cannot establish other ways of achieving intimacy, they may drift apart.

Divorce and Affairs

Dean and Ginger were each on the brink of an affair when they came for therapy. Backtracking to the origin of the problem, they both zeroed in on the Immersion phase of infertility. It was then that sex first become a "chore." Dean became a premature ejaculator[1] and Ginger felt that sex "was no longer sexy."

The loss of sexual attraction coupled with communication difficulties may lead to emotional distance, even alienation, in the Legacy years. This creates an atmosphere conducive to affairs.

Shelley and Richard came for therapy after Shelley found out that Richard was having an affair with a coworker. Each was caught up in the emotional upheaval of the affair, and the initial therapeutic focus was on the immediate crisis. However, after some of the dust had settled, and a couple history was taken, they were able to locate the seeds for the affair: infertility and its treatments 6 years before the affair was discovered. It was then that the partner's emotional detachment from each other had begun.

Each phase of infertility has its particular issues that might serve as the impetus for a divorce or an affair. For example, in Mobilization, a diagnosis of infertility may lead fertile partners to opt out of the marriage in search of a partner with whom to create a child. Whereas in other cultures, it is often expected that the fertile partner will annul or leave the marriage if there is no possibility of reproduction, in contemporary Western society, this is not culturally acceptable. Nevertheless, some may feel that if they are not able to have their own genetically related child, the marriage is no longer viable.

Once in Immersion, couples are so focused on medical treatment, even when conflict is great, it is unusual for either partner to initiate a

---

[1]Although the current medical nomenclature is "rapid ejaculation," "premature ejaculation" is the terminology most commonly used by both medical professionals and lay people.

divorce. However, if partners have turned to others outside the relationship for comfort and solace, the ensuing emotional distance can become the prologue to an affair. The roots of an affair may also be traced back to the Resolution phase. If couples are unable to come to terms with their infertility, mourn together, agree on their decisions regarding children, and plan their future lives, a significant disaffection may result. Consequently, they may be more susceptible to having an affair.

> Robert and Barbara came to therapy because she discovered he was having an affair. As partners in a successful computer consulting business, they were very well regarded in their field and had shared the rewarding experience of creating this business. However, after unsuccessful treatment for unexplained infertility, they realized that without children to raise—their "next project"—they had very little connection to each other. Feeling the marriage was over because they could not have a child, Robert left his wife to have an affair, hoping he could have a child with this other woman.

In Legacy, Couples who are unable to revive a satisfying sex life, or cannot find other ways to establish intimacy, may find that no matter how well they coped with their infertility their marriages seem empty.

THE INFERTILE IDENTITY

Although it is common for couples who had once considered themselves infertile and who later have children to retain scars from the infertile experience (Bernstein et al., 1988), for some, the fleeting involvement with infertility specialists seems like an insignificant part of their past.

> Alice and Edward had undergone 6 months of infertility treatments before the birth of their first child. "You know," said Alice, "I forgot all about it till just now. If Edward didn't mention it, I doubt I'd have remembered it. . . . I know I was diagnosed as having an infertility condition, but since I got pregnant and had a kid, I doubt that the doctors knew what they were talking about. . . . They could have been wrong." Edward said, "I don't think the doctors were wrong, but it was nothing of much significance in our lives."

For others who have had only brief encounters with infertility, the negative consequences are deeper and more long-lasting.

> Danielle and Ron also took only 6 months to get pregnant with their first child. But, "things were never quite the same afterward,"

said Ron. "When I got the results of the tests that showed a low sperm count, it shook me up. . . . It probably changed how I saw and see myself today." "I think we were both shaken by it," said Danielle. "They didn't treat it in any way, no inseminations and no hormones, just the diagnosis. . . . But it's one of those things in life that you only need to be close to for a very short time to feel changed. When I hear infertility mentioned on TV or the radio, I get a pang. . . . It feels like something's still wrong with me."

Couples who encounter infertility and then choose not to have children come face to face with an often disapproving, child-centered culture that views them as unusual at best and as abnormal or deviant at worst. In contemporary America, feminism notwithstanding, these couples, especially women, are likely to encounter implicit and explicit criticism. Although the greatest criticism may come shortly after their decision, in the words of one woman, it continues as "background noise" for years.

THE COUPLE AND THE SUPPORT SYSTEM

If a child has come into the family through donor conception or adoption, painful feelings about the infertility are often evoked at life-cycle events such as births, marriages, and deaths. These events can remind parents of the lack of the biological connection. Parents of donor-conceived or adopted children sometimes encounter differential treatment towards their child, by relatives who seem to value these children less than other children in the family. However, despite the objections relatives may have, most accept the child once he or she arrives.

Anita and Arnold had decided to try using donor eggs after tests showed that Anita was in early menopause. During Anita's pregnancy with twins, her parents were quite dubious about the process, and felt that Arnold's parents were the only "real" grandparents. However, after the twins were born, Anita's mother visited her every day to help out, and her father doted on the baby girls.

Couples without children may face the greatest burden in Legacy. Having a different status than their siblings with children, their families may never regard them as being truly adult. Even if a couple feels good about their decision, the culture reacts to them as a "childless couple" and they may be angry if people assume they could not have children rather than this being their choice.

In addition, as part of the "sandwich generation," baby boomers who do not have children may find themselves forced to care for aging parents. Siblings with children often assume that the lack of children makes it easier for the couple to drop everything and disrupt their lives to go to the hospital and so forth.

> Nicki was one of six children. Her mother was an alcoholic and periodically needed someone to rescue her when she was on a binge. Having no children, Nicki was usually elected.

PARENTING AFTER INFERTILITY

Couples who struggled with infertility often treasure their children with a greater sense of appreciation than those who had babies easily (Golombok, Cook, Bish, & Murray, 1995). For those who had to contend with infertility, the child may assume an almost sacred status.

Golombok et al. (1995) conducted a study of family adjustment after infertility, with four groups of subjects—families with a child aged 4–8, either (1) conceived naturally, (2) conceived by IVF, (3) conceived by DI, or (4) adopted. The researchers found that parents who had struggled with infertility showed greater warmth, emotional involvement, and parent–child interaction than parents of children conceived without difficulties. In addition, the latter couples had "a greater incidence of marital difficulties" and "higher levels of anxiety and depression" (p. 290). There were no significant differences in emotional, behavioral, or relationship adjustments among children who were conceived naturally, conceived with assisted reproduction, or adopted. Golombok et al. concluded that "the quality of parenting in families of a child conceived by assisted conception is *superior* to that shown by families with a naturally conceived child, *even when gamete donation is used in the child's conception*" [italics added] (p. 295).

In another study (Olivennes et al., 1997), 6- to 13-year-old children conceived by IVF had no higher incidence of psychosocial problems than average, and they were within the normal range compared with their peers in physical, intellectual, and psychological development.

An earlier study of 20 mothers who had conceived by IVF (Burns, 1990) reported different results: that these mothers may be overprotective, overindulgent, or abusive. Nearly 60% of the mothers classified themselves as "overprotective/child-centered" and 55% as "abusive/neglectful" whereas 30% of comparison subjects rated themselves as "overprotective/child-centered" and 20% as "abusive/neglectful" (Burns, 1990, p. 181). This study showed an increased incidence of psychosocial problems in both the IVF parents (e.g., depression, alcoholism, drug abuse) and children (e.g., school problems, identity issues, attention-deficit disorder, etc.). Burns also reported difficulties in bonding for 50% of these families.

The discrepancy between the two studies may be related to the degree to which these parents have resolved their feelings of infertility-related loss. Linda Salzer (1996), an adoption specialist, describes some of the reactions unresolved infertility can evoke in adoptive parents, which can also be applied to donor situations:

1. Continued denial of disappointment or grief; continuous sadness.
2. Frequent fantasies of an ideal biological child related to both parents.
3. Extreme fear that child will not live up to family standards.
4. Difficulty providing firm and effective discipline.
5. Discomfort in discussing or acknowledging the child's birth parent(s) (donor).
6. Overprotection or overcontrol of the child.
7. Keeping adoption (donor conception) a secret.
8. Extreme anxiety in discussing adoption (donor conception) with the child.
9. Excessive talking about adoption (donor conception).
10. Overly high expectations of oneself as a parent.

Candace had never sorted out her feelings about not having a genetically related child. When her adopted son, Jason, was diagnosed with a learning disability, she was unable to accept the diagnosis and insisted he was lazy. Her unresolved feelings about the infertility made it difficult for her to accept the child she had instead of the one she wished for. She enrolled him in her alma mater, a competitive school that stressed high achievement, even though he would have been better served at a school that was less academically demanding. He required a great deal of tutoring in order to keep him from failing. This added to his sense of difference and inadequacy.

Although research (Golombok et al., 1995; Olivennes, 1997) indicates that couples who have struggled with infertility tend to make better than average parents, some couples in the Infertility Project have talked about their difficulty setting limits, or becoming so invested in parenting that the couple's relationship suffered.

Gene and Laura had had three miscarriages and had been in infertility treatments for 2 years before they gave birth to Ashley.

Observing their interactions in a therapy session, it was clear that although Ashley played nicely by herself, the parents were distracted by what she was doing, continually jumping up and hovering over her. Although Ashley was in no danger, Gene kept putting his hand behind her head to prevent her from bumping it. He was aware and embarrassed that he was overprotective and acknowledged that it was because they had tried so hard to have the baby. "I know that sometimes I should let her cry," he said, "but I just can't help it. As soon as I hear her whimper, I have to go comfort her anyway."

Parents of donor-conceived or adopted children, may feel confused and guilty that they still mourn the loss of a biological child, and disloyal to the child they have.

Legacy and the Child

The literature on adopted children's attitudes toward adoption (Brinich, 1990), which we can assume applies to donor-conceived children as well, shows that children's feelings about the way they entered their family is strongly influenced by their parents' adjustment to and acceptance of their choice of how to create a family.

It has been speculated that children conceived with donor gametes may experience fewer losses than adopted children, in that they may feel they were always wanted rather than "given away," as many adopted children experience their adoptions. Nonetheless, both sets of children will have to contend with feelings of being "different" from others in terms of their origins.

Adoptive parents may be unaware of the losses and loyalty conflicts their children experience as part of adoption. As discussed earlier, closed adoption systems promote the belief that full membership in an adoptive family requires the relinquishment of all ties to the birth family. Similarly, adoptive parents may mistakenly believe that to love their adopted child, they should no longer think about the genetically related child they might have had or feel any of the losses of infertility. To do so feels disloyal to their adopted child, who, in turn, feels disloyal when feelings about the birth parents arise. The child often worries that if the adoptive parents knew how he or she felt, they would be hurt and the child would risk being rejected again.

As children tend to be concrete in their thinking, they deal with these loyalty struggles by defining one set of parents as the "good parents" and the other set of parents as the "bad parents." They may idealize their birth parents and demonize their adoptive parents or vice versa. During the developmental stage when many children fantasize that they are adopted, children who are in fact adopted may prolong this fantasy, maintaining the split between the "good" and "bad" parents (Sorosky, 1995, p. 139), and delay their ability to integrate their ambivalent feelings regarding both sets of parents.

In transracial and transcultural adoptions, children are at risk of losing their racial and cultural identity, and, with international adoptions, their connections to their country of origin. Many of these adopted children have grown up feeling "white," with little, if any, knowledge of, identification with, and pride in their heritage and culture. As they become young adults and experience society's stereotyping of and discrimination against them, they have few resources to deal with the racism they encounter. Not having learned to deal with this as young children, they personalize others' reactions to them and may feel bad about themselves.

How children cope with any differences between themselves and others depends on each child's temperament and resiliency. Those who want to conform may have a harder time than those who use their differences to feel unique and special.

> Linda, an adopted Korean girl, was one of a few Asian students in her high school. She enjoyed being unique and accentuated it by dressing in an offbeat way, highlighting her Asian heritage and her differences.

At times, an adopted child can feel that he or she is the adoptive parents' "second choice"; had they been able to get pregnant and have the child they *really* wanted, "I wouldn't be here." These children carry within them the "ghost" (Lifton, 1988) of the child their adoptive parents could have had, and fear that they will never measure up. Adopted children can also feel that they were "dropped"—as though into thin air—by their birth parents and "saved" from abandonment by their adoptive parents. These children may consciously or unconsciously fear that their adoptive parents might also "give them up." These fears may be expressed through an adopted child's compliance ("I had better be perfect so as not to disappoint them") or through his or her rebellion ("I will never match up, so why try?").

In addition, young children are naturally egocentric, believing that everything that happens is because of them. It is common for adopted children to believe, at some stage in their understanding the "whys" of adoption, that it was something in them that was lacking or "bad" that caused the birth parents to "give them up." Having already "lost" one family— the birth parents—adopted children can be sensitive to issues of loss.

If parents subtly (or overtly) prohibit expressions of curiosity or sadness, the child's ability to process his or her own grief is thwarted. This can be the most damaging aspect of adoption for the child, as parents are the child's primary resource to deal with these issues, and children depend on parents to help them figure out the central question for all adoptees, "Why was I given up?" Without their adoptive parents' support, even when these children become adults and decide to search for their birth parents, they do not share their search with their adoptive parents or they undertake a search only after their adoptive parents have died.

The most beneficial legacies for adoptive families are ones in which the parents create a loving atmosphere where adoption is discussed openly as something in which all have participated, and everyone feels comfortable expressing their feelings about it. This allows children to feel free to love both sets of parents and families and to grieve the losses that are inherent in adoption.

Disclosure

During Legacy, parents of donor and adopted children face the task of talking with their children about their origins. Although years of adoption research have concluded that full disclosure is best for the child and family (Brinich, 1990; Hartman, 1993), donor-conceived children have not been studied long and thoroughly enough for any similar assertion. Some writers (e.g., Lieber Wilkins, 1995; Baran & Pannor, 1989) believe that children have the right to know about their genetic heritage. In practice, parents who reveal information about the donor (or, indeed, any other ART conception) to their children are rare (Golombok et al., 1995; Greenfeld, 1995). Couples may be waiting until their children are older to discuss ART or donor conception, thinking or believing it will be easier for their children to understand. However, delaying telling can cause other problems. Even when both parents' genes are involved, the story of the child's conception can engender feelings of difference or shame.

> At the age of 8 years, one IVF-conceived child became curious about reproduction. Assuming this would be an easy discussion, her parents told her the details of her conception. They were surprised at the intensity of her reaction to learning she was conceived in a petri dish. She exclaimed, "I feel crooked. I wasn't inside Mommy all the time."

Disclosure raises complicated issues. Sometimes parents may tell their children once or twice and then convey the message that the subject is closed, or they may feel too threatened to discuss it and decide to avoid it altogether. For parents of donor-conceived or adopted children, fearful of rejection or insecure about their role, questions about their place in the child's life may arise: What is their role with the child to be? What will the child think when he or she finds out?

Sometimes, fear of the negative reactions of others keeps parents from telling their child about his or her donor conception. Parents' perception of stigma, however, can depend on their social context, particularly with egg donation because it is so new. In families in which there was disagreement about infertility treatments, disclosure may bring up all the old resentments, as well as any feelings they may have toward the children as a result of these resentments. Parents whose sense of shame is compounded by problematic family of origin legacies, may feel, for example, that their infertility "proves" that they are not entitled to their child's love, and disclosure may be particularly threatening for them.

SECONDARY INFERTILITY

In Legacy, couples who experienced secondary infertility may confront issues discussed in earlier phases, for example, loss of their ideal family size and dealing with intrusive questions. They may also feel that only having one child makes that child too "precious." The potential loss of that child would mean the loss of parenthood completely.

> Leonora was preparing for a tubal ligation when her 7-year-old daughter was rushed to the hospital with a life-threatening condition. It was touch and go all night, and Leonora found herself thinking that although she would be devastated if her daughter died, she could have another child. The daughter survived, but Leonora decided to postpone having the tubal ligation. Her friend, Roberta, whose secondary infertility prevented her from having a second child, lived through a similar scare with her son, but felt the ordeal was doubly difficult: "I would lose everything."

For couples with secondary infertility, perhaps the greatest challenge in Legacy is integrating a donor-conceived or adopted child into a family with an existing child who is genetically related to both parents. Popular mythology has generated the belief that in these families, the biological child is given preferential treatment. In reality, parents in these situations may become protective of the adopted or donor-conceived child, seeing him or her as "the miracle child." However, when parents are so solicitous, the child can easily feel singled out.

Because sibling rivalry is present in many families, how each child enters the family often becomes ammunition in sibling struggles.

There might be a significant gap in ages between the children, or there may be considerable differences in physical appearance. However, it is important to bear in mind, as with other issues connected to the child's origins, handling these differences can be hampered by parents' lingering negative feelings about their infertility.

> In one Caucasian family with secondary infertility, the youngest was a biracial child and clearly different from her sibling. The parents acted as though they were one big happy family and that differences did not exist. They came to therapy because the adopted child was depressed and performing below grade-level schoolwork. As therapy progressed, it became clear that she was uncomfortable with this pretense. "Everybody on the street looks at us like I'm different, like, 'What's with this family? White parents, white kid, and black kid?' but my parents act like it's not happening," she said.

For families who have struggled with secondary infertility and choose to increase their family through the use of donor gametes, they have the luxury of disclosing this information if, when, and to whom they choose. Regardless of whether they have used a sperm or egg donor, the fact that the woman carries the pregnancy allows for a privacy adoptive parents do not have. Unfortunately, if these parents choose to maintain secrecy around their child's conception, there may be potentially negative consequences in the future.

Decision making around disclosure can present a real challenge for couples who have had children through the use of donors, particularly when partners are polarized in their preferences. As yet untested are the effects that may ensue from only one parent being genetically related to the child, which can affect the couple's relationship as well as the relationship between each parent and the child. Keeping the donor conception a secret increases the potential explosiveness of the situation as secrets become ammunition if partners become adversaries.

Methods for dealing with these issues as they arise in therapy will be addressed in the next chapter.

14

⌒

THERAPEUTIC APPROACH
IN THE LEGACY PHASE

"I see us as postfertile with a child and a life, not the
way we hoped but a blessing anyway. For my wife,
infertility never seems to go away. She's always aware of
how many children other couples have. The essential
difference is that I see infertility as part of the past, and
she sees it as an endless present."

Although many couples report that the reverberations of infertility continue long into the future, clinicians can, nonetheless, intervene to minimize problematic legacies. Therapeutic intervention can help couples
turn this difficult event into an opportunity to enhance their relationships.

Because infertility is typically a dark and painful chapter in a couple's life, they often avoid talking about it, creating legacies that are
often covert. As a result, a couple's past experience with infertility is
rarely raised when presenting for treatment. As we became more sensi-
tized to the problematic legacies of infertility through our work in the
Project, we began to ask the couples in our practices about a history of
infertility. We found it was far more prevalent and problematic than we
had previously thought.

PRESENTING PROBLEM

In the Legacy phase, couples rarely seek treatment because of past problems with infertility, as they are not likely to consider the relevance of their current difficulties to infertility. Instead, they are likely to seek therapy for a variety of relational difficulties which may or may not be related to the couple's past encounter with infertility.

RESPECT AND LIMIT THE INFLUENCE OF INFERTILITY

If infertility surfaces in the course of taking the couple's history, the clinician can ask how the couple weathered the ordeal. He or she may also acknowledge the impact of infertility by saying many couples experience it as a major life crisis that can be as traumatic as divorce or the death of a child (Humphrey, 1986). It is important to acknowledge that it was a powerful event in their lives, although most couples need little reminder of their suffering. By recognizing infertility's power, the couple may make a connection between infertility and their current distress, and appreciate their accomplishment in having survived this ordeal.

Often, couples are disturbed to find that the infertility is still affecting them. If this is so, the clinician can ask about their painful feelings related to the infertility, specifically about whether there have been special moments when these feelings are likely to occur. Normalizing their lingering feelings of loss allows them to feel more comfortable when discussing infertility's impact. It may be helpful to probe each partner's ability to communicate with the other when these painful feelings arise. The following kinds of questions are suggestive of how to explore this area:

- Are there times you still think about the infertility?
- Do you share those moments with each other?
- When was the last time the two of you discussed the infertility?
- What worries do each of you have about sharing your feelings about the infertility?

THE THERAPIST'S ROLE

As in all phases, a therapist must be careful to examine his or her personal feelings about reproductive choices in order to avoid making assumptions about couples or imposing his or her own attitudes. If the

clinician believes that in having a child the legacies of infertility are ame-
liorated, he or she may fail to understand the depth of a couple's distress.

A clinician might also assume that couples who do not have children are either selfish and self-centered or deprived. In order to understand the couple's experience, the therapist can ask, "When you first got
together did you plan to have children?"

If the therapist is biased toward adoption or believes in letting
nature take its course, he or she might disapprove of the large sums of
money spent on infertility treatments, or think that couples who adopt
are more selfless and thus admirable. Furthermore, the therapist might
be less able to understand the distress associated with failed medical
treatments.

Therapists need to be aware of the powerful impact of infertility
and not to assume it is past history with little emotional charge in the
present.

> Long after her encounter with infertility, Renee realized that she
> avoided serving on committees in her children's school because she
> felt "less able, less normal, less entitled" than other mothers; she
> traced the start of these feelings to the infertility.

Once again, with increased awareness of personal biases, the clinician is
best able to track how couples responded to their infertility, how each
partner coped, and what impact it had on the relationship.

The following questions will help the therapist examine his or her
biases on these issues:

- What values and beliefs do I have about the meaning and value
  of children?
- What views do I have about family size?
- Do I tend to underemphasize the infertility? Or do I overempha-
  size the infertility?
- Do I assume a child is the antidote to all of the sadness?

Eliciting the Story

Therapists who work with couples in the Legacy phase need to ask
about a history of infertility. Couples may have endured a poor sexual
relationship or conflicts in communication for years without connecting
these problems to their failed attempts to get pregnant.

In using a genogram, a history of infertility can be discovered
(McGoldrick & Gerson, 1985). A genogram may reveal a significant

period of time from the marriage to the birth of the first child, and large gaps in age between the children. The following questions can elicit the history of infertility and its effects:

> Was it your choice not to have children?
>
> Are you satisfied with the size of your family?
>
> Which one of you has been most disappointed with not having (or not having more) children?
>
> If infertility is the reason you have no children, or only one child, do you think it has had an impact on your relationship? If so, how?
>
> Is there any part of the current problem that may be related to the infertility?
>
> Are there any positive changes in the relationship as the result of the infertility?

WORKING WITH THE COUPLE: THERAPEUTIC ISSUES, TECHNIQUES, AND STRATEGIES

There are several ways of understanding how infertility has affected the couple. Has it put distance between partners? Are there unresolved problems, unspoken resentments, or disappointments? Or has the ordeal made the relationship stronger? If there were no children, the therapist can look at how partners restructured their lives and whether they have been able to put their energies into other endeavors.

Because couples who have been unable to have children often take on a nurturing, mentoring role in their community, the clinician can broach this possibility with couples who have been unable to satisfy these goals:

- Has the meaning and value of children changed for you because of the infertility experience?
- What about parenting was important to you?
- Have you been able to fill some of the needs in ways other than having children?
- [When couples talk about the wish to leave a lasting legacy] Do you think it is worth exploring some other way of leaving your mark?

Communication Gaps

During the prolonged period of stress and sadness, some partners may have lost all desire to communicate with each other. In the Legacy phase, ruptures may be evident in a couple's relationship ranging from open hostility to living separate lives.

Often people are so entrenched in unresolved, undiscussed problems that they cannot see a way out of the morass. Asking questions about the past can remind couples of when life was better and why they chose each other. Future questions (Penn, 1985) such as "In a year from now if this resentment is no longer part of your lives, where would you like your relationship to be going?" can suggest the possibility of a future life liberated from past resentments.

A focus solely on improving communication skills may be insufficient for couples who are still holding onto past resentments. For these couples, clinicians can serve as facilitators in guiding couples through a discussion of the past. The process can be started with questions such as "Have you ever discussed what infertility has meant to each of you?"

Once a history of infertility is established, the therapist can normalize the nature of their experience and their inclination to distance from it. The clinician can suggest that it is worthwhile to review their experiences so that each may learn more about the other partner's thoughts and feelings at that time. Sometimes significant concerns have not been discussed, and it can be useful to raise them now.

> Tammy and Craig were in their 40s and had been dating for 10 years prior to marriage. When Tammy was 39, she had become pregnant and had had an abortion because Craig was adamantly opposed to having a child. When they tried to conceive after they were married, Tammy was diagnosed with "old eggs" after two miscarriages.
>
> When they came for therapy several years later, although they had adopted a son who was thriving and whom they dearly loved, Tammy revealed in a separate session that she was still furious with Craig: "He wasted my childbearing years." She felt that she could not say this to him because "I'm fearful of upsetting the only adult with whom I've created a sense of family, a sense of having a future together, my main connection in life." The therapist asked, "What's your fear? Why do you think Craig needs the protection? Why are you so afraid of upsetting him?" Tammy responded, "He gets defensive, angry, says 'I did my best, I've had enough. What's the point of wallowing in it?' And, I think I agree. I hate myself for still being here, but I also hate him." The therapist introduced the idea that perhaps Craig himself regretted how he had acted in the past, and wondered if Tammy would invite Craig to come for a few sessions to talk about the unhappiness between them over the past. Tammy needed to stop protecting Craig from her distress, and Craig needed to feel there was a way to end the impasse without feeling blamed.

In therapy, they explored how to separate the Craig of today from the younger Craig of the past, and to understand the context in which his past choices were made. He was able to talk about his chronic doubts about having the capacity to be a person on whom others might rely. Having now proved himself as a husband, a father, and a professional, he currently saw himself as having changed from the man he was. As this capable partner, distinct from the insecure younger person of himself, he was able to understand Tammy's feelings about the past, and her grief about not experiencing pregnancy and childbirth. Through this therapy, they came to understand that in the future there would likely be periodic moments of sadness and remorse. In therapy, they were able to talk about how to cope with these feelings and each other at those times. They worked out signals, specific ways each might let the other know it was time to recognize and deal with a spillover from the past: What might she say? How could he listen? What would comfort her? Him? How would she let him know when an episode was over? How would they return to life again? In the process of rehearsing how to handle these issues in the future, they began to talk more openly about the infertility. She cried, and he comforted her. Then, unexpectedly, Craig began to sob almost uncontrollably. He talked about the child he had "lost" and the feeling that he had broken his generational line. Tammy was able to comfort him and join him in his grief—a mutual mourning process that had never occurred before.

Revitalizing Sex

Couples usually enter therapy because of intimacy problems, not sexual problems. This larger problem may stem from the infertility and the way in which decisions were made and partners treated each other at the time. It can be useful to explore those decisions and what the partners' responses to each other were during the earlier phases of infertility. As mentioned, it is difficult to maintain intimacy when sex no longer serves as a physical counterpart to emotional closeness.

Although sexual problems that have persisted for a long time are hard to address when partners believe that their sexual attraction to each other has been lost forever, even partners who feel the spark is retrievable may be unable to rekindle it. Therefore, sexual activities might be presented as "experiments"; this way, if couples encounter little success in such endeavors, they are less likely to feel that they have failed, adding yet another negative story to the legacy of infertility.

Even if the couple is aware of the paradox of trying to have a spontaneous, pleasurable sexual relationship while desperate to get pregnant, and understand how the baby-making agenda affected their sexual enjoyment, they may need to be reminded that this was the unfortunate fall-out from the infertility rather than the "fault" or lack of desirability of either partner. When the problem is externalized in this way, the clinician can follow with questions such as "How are you two going to reclaim the fun in sex that you had before the infertility?" The revitalization of the couple's sex life can be posed as a mutual project in which the remedial strategies of sex therapies can be assigned as at-home exercises. The clinician can suggest playful and sensual activities to see whether their sexual lives together can be reclaimed. The following are several standard techniques we have used:

• Introduce the idea of novelty. Suggest making love away from the marital bed where they tried to conceive the baby or where they have experienced many sexual failures. The therapist can suggest having a romantic dinner, and then making love in any room but the bedroom.
• Suggest that the partners learn what feels good for themselves and each other through sensual massage.
• If they have no religious or ethical objection, propose that they might use erotic videos or magazines together. Most couples feel some embarrassment about exploring eroticism but are also curious. Therefore, they may feel more comfortable with the idea if it is posed by the clinician.
• Clarify when physical affection is a signal for cuddling or a signal for sex. Sometimes when couples are having sexual problems, they avoid all physical contact for fear it will be interpreted as a sexual overture. Partners are often able to salvage their physical closeness when they discuss the distinction, and get better at signaling and reading each other's physical gestures. It is important to emphasize the need to separate the two kinds of physicality—just a hug or a hug as a prologue to sexual activity. Paradoxically, once couples feel the safety of "just cuddling," they often feel closer to each other and more willing, on other occasions, to engage in love-making "experiments."

When sexual problems are longstanding and entrenched, they may not shift in spite of uncovering the problematic patterns that developed during the infertility. In these cases, the clinician can prescribe sensate focus exercises or refer the couple for sex therapy.

EXPLORE COUPLES' BELIEF SYSTEMS

The beliefs to be explored during Legacy are similar to those in other phases. Here, the emphasis is on finding the long-term impact that infertility has had on each partner and the couple. Although this varies from person to person, nearly everyone is left with negative imprints on how they see themselves as individuals and as a couple. Couple therapy undertaken during Legacy provides an opportunity to modify the negative images and highlight the beneficial ones.

The first step is to ask the couple about whether and how their infertility may have changed the ways they saw themselves and their relationship. The second is to explore the cultural, familial, and personal contexts from which they drew their conclusions. As a third step, couples can be invited to modify these perceptions. Before proceeding in this direction, it is important to temper one's therapeutic zeal with the "reminder" that infertility's impact is so profound and tenacious that efforts to counteract its effects are difficult, and can take considerable time and effort.

As mentioned in earlier chapters, infertility often gives rise to fatalistic world views such as "Bad things always happen to me." In Legacy, these perspectives may have become organizing principles, which can be reinforced by subsequent adversities. The therapist can explore these world views with the couple:

- What ideas about infertility did you have as you were experiencing it?
- Have those changed as time has gone by?
- What would happen if you decided to let go of these ideas?
- Which of you would be most likely to let go?
- What would happen if you had a different idea?
- How might your life change?
- Did you have other kinds of ideas before the infertility?

Because the inability to reproduce raises questions about one's sexuality, potency, and attractiveness, it is helpful to stress that although our culture conflates sexuality and fertility, the two are distinct. Depending on the couple, the clinician may decide that it is preferable to discuss sexual legacies in separate sessions. This is particularly applicable when discussing each partner's feelings about the other. The following questions can be asked in either individual or couple sessions:

- Do you see yourself as any less sexy as a woman/man because you were unable to produce a baby? If so, where did you learn that?
- Can you think of any advantage to figuring out how to see yourself as sexy even though you could not produce a child?

FACILITATE MOURNING

Some people come from a background in which there was relative ease in talking about loss and death, whereas in other families these subjects are taboo. To assess whether couples have sufficiently dealt with the losses of infertility, the clinician may want to open a discussion about the couple's comfort with discussing and dealing with loss:

- How have your families dealt with loss and the expression of grief?
- How comfortable were your families in talking about death?
- Do you think this pattern has influenced the way you handle your sad feelings?

Exploring these issues not only reveals possible impediments to grieving, it also provides couples with an opportunity to mourn the losses of infertility together.

As in earlier phases, clinicians can suggest that couples may wish to acknowledge more formally the child that never was and mourn that loss. The following is the text of a ritual, which was part of the couple's therapy, in which they commemorated a child lost in miscarriage.

Requiem for a Small Bubak[1]

"Small Bubak. On this day, we light a candle for you.

"We conceived you in April. You were made out of our love and hope. We wanted to be parents. We wanted to create a life that we could love and nourish. We wanted to see a more perfect version of ourselves. We wanted to create an us. We wanted to heal our childhood wounds and have the family we never had.

"As you grew, our excitement rose. We faced our fears of parenthood, our anxieties of inadequacy, and our loss of control. We could feel you kick. We looked forward to your life. We were ready to be parents.

"We remembered your sister, who died last year. She was gone before we could give her a name. She drowned in blood just days after our wedding.

"We took you to Provincetown, walked in the sand, enjoyed the sun. We didn't know you would leave us so soon.

"On Friday, you were fine. But, on Monday, the cervix began to

---

[1]Bubak is a Czech mythical character known for his grumpiness. Eugene Ward, who wrote the requiem, used Bubak as a term of endearment. Reprinted by permission.

open. And our lives began to close. The doctor could not stop you. The Ritadrine could not stop you, Our tears could not stop you.

"You were born alive, doomed to a moment's life, a meteor that crashed into our hearts. We cried and screamed, pleading and begging for your life. But you did not hear us.

"We could not forgive you then. And when your brother died, he was another casualty of the blood. We had only our imperfect selves, our pain and disappointment. Our hope for a child, the bridge of love and life between us was broken. We became lost in our sorrows and we were bathed in bitterness.

"Our hearts are heavy still. Our losses weigh heavily on us. We wonder why we have been denied the gift of life. And yet we live on together.

"We wish you were here. We love you. We forgive you. We will never forget you. With our breath, we set you free."

EXPLORE PARENT–CHILD RELATIONSHIP

Many of the couples who came to a posttherapy follow-up session were concerned about being overprotective with their children. We do not assume that overprotection is more of an issue after infertility, and we cannot infer that these parents are more worried about being overprotective than other new parents. Yet it is still a concern worth raising and discussing in therapy.

Couples whose children were conceived with a donor may feel imbalances in their relationship with their child, which can take many forms. The following example illustrates both overprotection and donor imbalances:

> Sid and Deborah's daughter was conceived through the use of donor sperm. In therapy around child-focused problems, it became clear that although they differed in their parenting styles, Sid always deferred to Deborah. The therapist asked if this was their style in other areas of their life, and each immediately said "No."
>
> The therapist then asked Sid if he thought he would defer to Deborah in terms of parenting if he and his daughter were genetically related. Sid quickly responded "No. I'm pretty sure I would hold firm to my opinion because I would feel she was mine as much as Deborah's."

Clinicians may be uncomfortable asking questions about how the differences in parents' genetic relationship to a child affects their parenting. However, it is important to acknowledge that this is not a legitimate criteria for feeling entitled to parent.

Disclosure

Much of what we know about the importance of disclosure comes from the field of adoption (Melina, 1989; Watkins & Fisher, 1993). It is clear that children who are not told of their adoption by their adoptive parents, and who find out from others, struggle with tremendous feelings of betrayal and distrust toward their adoptive parents. It remains to be seen whether research on the outcome of disclosure and nondisclosure on donor offspring will corroborate the findings of adoption.

Despite good intentions, many parents are uncomfortable raising the topics of ART, donor conception, or adoption when their child reaches the age they had deemed appropriate to initiate these discussions. The following is a common scenario regarding adoption disclosure:

> Brendan and Julie had always planned to tell their son, Liam, about his adoption. They knew exactly what they wanted to say and had rehearsed it many times before he was 2 years old. However, they found that once he was verbal and could understand what they were saying, they raised the topic of adoption less and less. They convinced themselves that because he was not asking questions, he must be comfortable with his adoptive status and that there was no need for them continually to "hammer him over the head" with the topic.

The literature on adoption indicates that parental reluctance to disclose adoption to children can be based on parents' negative and unresolved feelings about their infertility, their concerns that their child will be damaged or traumatized by the information, or their worries that when their child understands what it means to be adopted, he or she will love them less or believe that they love him or her less. In addition, parents may be concerned about the reactions of others when their child shares the story of his or her origins. Given the scant research on disclosure with donor conception, one can only speculate on the reasons parents might be reluctant to tell their children about their conception with donor gametes. In situations like these, it is crucial for the clinician to help couples understand the basis for their apprehensions and fears. Therapists working with these parents need to make room for these feelings, to normalize them, and to encourage couples to embrace them. Parents can love their child, *and* they can feel sad about the child they were not able to have. Giving expression to the sadness does not lessen their love, but may allow it to exist in an atmosphere free of guilt and shame. The therapist can normalize these concerns and remind the couples that their child's bonds and attachments to them are more secure than they believe.

However, the ability of partners to accept this reality may hinge on any persistent negative legacies associated with the infertility or the particular choice they made about how to become parents. In order to locate these problematic legacies, a variety of questions can be asked:

- Which one of you is more reluctant to discuss adoption (donor conception) with your child?
- What concerns do you each have about your child's understanding his or her origins?
- Why do you think that is? Why do you think your partner has such a hard time with it?
- What do you think would happen if you said more?
- Which of you worries more about the effects of disclosure, or nondisclosure, on your child?

When a couple is uneasy talking with their child about adoption or donor conception, the clinician can increase their comfort, first by discussing any lingering problematic legacies around infertility, then exploring specific fantasies and worries about telling the child, and finally explaining the benefits of disclosure to them and their child.

When to Tell

In the field of adoption, there is virtually no debate about *whether* children should be told of their adoption and little, if any, debate on *when* children should be told. Adoption literature has taught us that when children grow up "always knowing" of their adoptions, never remembering a specific time when they were told, the information becomes part of their "life or adoption story" and is eventually integrated into the adopted child's sense of self. As mentioned, this is not the case when adoptees learn of their adoptions from persons other than their adoptive parents or are told by their adoptive parents when they are older. In these unfortunate situations, adoptees are left confused and disoriented. A basic trust has been broken, a cornerstone—if not the foundation—of the adoptee's life must be questioned and reviewed (Watkins & Fisher, 1993).

When it comes to disclosure with the use of donor gametes, there is little research on when and whether to tell children of their donor conception. Although a few professionals contend that children do not need to know that donor gametes are part of their conception, most of the debate centers on the best age for children to be told of their donor conception. There are those (Baran & Pannor, 1989; Sorosky, 1995) who hold that donor conception is more complex than adoption and harder for children to understand. Therefore, these writers suggest withholding the information until a child is 9 or 10 years of age and is better able to understand the complexities involved.

However, given that no hard data exist on the best age to disclose donor conception to children, many professionals are applying what is known from the field of adoption to families parenting donor children, that it is best for children to be told at younger ages and to grow up "always knowing" (Lieber Wilkins, 1995), in spite of the fact that they are not cognitively capable of understanding the information. At an early age, they can hear the information as part of the story of how their family was formed, without attaching judgments or the sense of being different.

How to Talk with Children about Their Beginnings

The adoption literature advises parents to begin talking about adoption when their children are toddlers and to continue the discussions over the life of the family. Adoption disclosure is not a one-time event, but a process through which children come to understand what happened to them and why (Grotevant & McRoy, 1990; Melina, 1989). Clinicians must remind adoptive parents that in order to convey to their child that it is safe to talk about adoption, they must raise the subject and talk about it themselves.

> Ann and Bruce determined that their adopted daughter, Sofia, would grow up always knowing that her birth mother, Karen, cared about her and that they cared about Karen. One of the ways they did this was to mention Karen on Sofia's birthday every year and to comment on what Karen might be feeling and doing on this special day. In this indirect way, they let Sofia know they were comfortable talking about Karen.

Waiting for an adopted child to ask questions or pumping them for information with questions such as "Do you think about your birth mother?" can communicate that parents are not comfortable discussing the topic, and furthermore, that adoption is only the child's issue. The clinician can point out that adoption is a family matter and adopting a child creates an *adoptive family,* it does not create parents with an adopted child. It is important for parents to realize that children learn quickly that the topics permissible for discussion are those that are discussed with comfort. It is not enough to tell a child to "feel free to ask me any questions" and leave it at that. Parents need to discuss the matter openly and regularly. Otherwise, the child may hesitate to ask questions about his or her origins because he or she perceives the subject as being too difficult and painful for the adoptive parents to discuss.

Sometimes adoptive parents perceive their child's silence as indicating that the child is comfortable with what he or she has been told and has no "problems" with being adopted or is not interested in the subject. However, the clinician can inform them that adopted adults have taught us that for every question they asked their adoptive parents, there were 99 questions they were reluctant to ask.

Similar to talking to children about the "facts of life," sharing the adoption story is a process in which the story is told and retold, shaped and reshaped, and embellished with additional and specific information over time as the child matures and is able to understand the information intellectually and cognitively. Parents who are relatively comfortable with disclosure often start talking to their child when he or she is an infant in order to practice saying things they fear will be difficult to say or hurtful for the child to hear. The adoption story is central in the life of the adoptive family and over time should include answers to the following questions:

- Where did the baby come from?
- Who are the birth parents (including the birth father at some point)?
- What were the circumstances around the birth?
- Why did the birth parents relinquish the baby? Why was the baby placed in adoption?
- Why did the adoptive parents adopt (infertility)?
- How did the child and family get together?

With young children who have been adopted domestically, the adoption story can go something like this:

> "We wanted to be a mommy and daddy very much and tried very hard to make a baby grow inside Mommy's womb, but no baby grew there. After trying for a long time, we realized we didn't need to make a baby grow inside Mommy's womb to be parents; we could adopt. So we found a lady who had a baby growing in her womb. Guess who that baby was—you! But she didn't feel she could be a mommy to any baby at that time. She wanted you to

have a mommy and daddy who would take care of you and love you forever. We were all so happy when we met, and when you were born (and you were born just like everyone else in the world is born), we adopted you and took you home to be our baby FOR-EVER!!"

In situations involving international adoptions or the adoption of foster children, the story can be modified to fit each family's specific situation.

Because there is little research about whether, when, or how to tell donor conceived children about their origins, one can borrow from the adoption experience and literature. In the book *Mommy, Did I Grow in Your Tummy?* (Gordon, 1992), the author suggests that what is most important to children is to feel loved and wanted and to know that their parents have been honest with them about their beginnings. Gordon also provides suggestions for explaining complicated reproductive methods to young children who were conceived through the use of IVF, egg or sperm donors, or surrogates, or who were adopted. For example, in order to describe egg donation to a child, parents must first explain that all babies are made with sperm from a man and an egg from a woman. The author then suggests explaining it to children in the following way:

> A mom might not have an egg to join with the dad's sperm. But she can still grow a baby in her body. When this happens, another woman, called an *egg donor,* can help by donating or giving her eggs to meet and join with the dad's sperm. The doctor puts the donated egg and the dad's sperm into the mom so she can grow the baby. (Gordon, 1992, p. 19)

Couple Issues in Secondary Infertility

Blending a donor-conceived or adopted child into a family with existing genetically related children presents specific challenges, such as dealing with the adopted or donor-conceived child's possible feelings of being second best. Along with many other issues, children often use the ways they entered the family as ammunition in their ongoing sibling rivalries. At a workshop on raising adopted and biological siblings, a mother told this story:

> "I was in the kitchen and overheard my children arguing over who was loved more. When I heard my first child say, 'They love me more; they gave birth to me,' I shuddered and wanted to run into the room to protect my adopted child's feelings. When I heard him respond, 'They love me more; they paid more money for me,' I knew he needed no protection."

We know from adoption that it is important for families to celebrate all the ways that children join their families. It seems to follow that this would apply to all families in which the children have various genetic backgrounds, including all the possible combinations of donor-conceived, adopted, and jointly conceived children. It is just as important to tell the adoption or donor story as to tell about rushing to the hospital to give birth. Many adoptive families develop rituals to celebrate their "anniversary" date, the day the child and family came together, which can be a different date from the child's birthday. Adoption or "gotcha" day celebrations are examples of these kinds of rites. Ironically, often the nonadopted child feels envious that his or her adopted sibling gets two celebrations while he or she *only* celebrates his or her birthday.

LEGACY IS ONGOING

Clinicians are often unaware of the depth of despair couples have experienced because of infertility. As a result, they do not consider infertility's lasting legacies or routinely inquire about it when taking family histories. Infertility can be a significant factor in the formation of a couples' presenting problems, even though it predated therapy by many years. Therefore, history taking can be a spring-board to unearthing the legacies of infertility, and, because such legacies are enduring and malleable, they can be explored at any time.

15

⊷

CONCLUSION

The prospect of childlessness for couples who want to have children throws lives into chaos and places relationships in jeopardy. Infertility, a continuing ordeal that is permeated with loss, and one in which fundamental assumptions about life, sexual identity, social roles, marriage, and parenthood are turned topsy-turvy, is also a time in which couples must make medical decisions that will have enduring consequences. No matter what the outcome is in regard to children, the ordeal of infertility reverberates long after the couple leaves the medical arena. If there are children, they too may inherit the legacies of infertility.

Medicine, with its ever-expanding field of assisted reproductive technologies, offers the promise of a child. Unfortunately, each new protocol may have the effect of prolonging the time a couple spends involved in treatment. And, because failures are common during the treatment-focused phase, a couple is likely to experience protracted periods of acute distress. Furthermore, many of the latest emerging infertility procedures present additional problems of their own. The increasing availability of third-party protocols such as gamete donation (especially egg) and surrogacy means that an increasing number of families (parents, children, and perhaps donors) will be trying to cope with a variety of complex and confusing issues.

As the population of couples postponing childbearing grows, therapists can expect to see more and more couples who struggle with infertility. In the coming years, we are also likely to see a continuing flow of extraordinary reproductive technologies that will, no doubt, raise perplexing psychological, legal, social, and ethical questions. Human cloning, for example, may be just such a possibility. While ethicists, social scientists, and attorneys debate these issues, couples will likely be consulting with clinicians about their situations and the decisions they face.

We believe that many couples who will be struggling with infertility can benefit from the assistance of clinicians who are familiar with the material covered in our text—namely, the phases of infertility, the themes that are likely to arise, and the relevant therapeutic interventions. By helping couples to think through their experiences, understand their feelings, and make wise decisions, clinicians can help couples negotiate the landscape of infertility

Finally, in the course of our research, our meetings with couples, and the writing of this book, we have each been forced to examine a host of assumptions, attitudes, and feelings about infertility and its treatments. The reader may find him- or herself in a similar position. Although this can be an unsettling process, we have each found it to be as valuable personally as it is beneficial to the couples with whom we work.

Appendix

MEDICAL EVALUATION AND TREATMENT OF INFERTILITY: A BRIEF GUIDE FOR CLINICIANS

Because medical treatments lie at the center of the infertility experience, familiarity with medical diagnostic and treatment procedures is essential for clinicians who work with couples who struggle with infertility. The following brief overview of diagnostic and treatment protocols was excerpted from *The Couple's Guide to Fertility* (revised edition; Berger et al., 1995) and *Dr. Richard Marrs' Fertility Book* (Marrs, 1997).

OVERVIEW OF REPRODUCTION

Reproduction is a complex, multifaceted process that begins in the brain where males and females initiate a chain of hormonal secretions that lead to ovulation and sperm production. The hypothalamus secretes gonadotropin-releasing hormone (GnRH), which stimulates the pituitary gland to produce luteinizing hormone (LH) and follicle-stimulating hormone (FSH). These, in turn, target the reproductive organs and stimulate sperm production and ovulation.

Men's reproductive mechanism proceeds as follows: After sperm are produced, during ejaculation they travel from the testicles through the epididymis and vas deferens to the urethra, where the sperm combines with semen produced by the seminal vesicles and prostate gland. Sperm, ejaculated into the vagina, travel through the cervix, uterus, and fallopian tubes in search of eggs. When and if sperm encounter an egg, they surround it and one sperm penetrates the egg, while the egg instantly alters its outer wall (the zona pellucida) so that it is impenetrable by other sperm.

Women's reproductive process is somewhat more complex: FSH stimulates follicles in the ovaries to produce eggs. Normally the ovaries alternate monthly in egg production, and only one egg out of the several maturing eggs is actually released. LH triggers the release of the egg, which is then "scooped up" by the tiny finger-like projections at the end of the fallopian tube (fimbria). The cilia in the fallopian tube move the egg toward the uterus, where it may encounter and be fertilized by a sperm cell. At the time of ovulation, when fertility is at its highest, the woman's cervical mucus becomes thin and of an egg-white consistency; the mucus helps sperm to survive and facilitates its travel toward the egg. At other times, the mucus is thick, cloudy, and hard to penetrate. When an egg is released, the corpus luteum forms at the collapsed follicle and produces progesterone, which signals the uterus to prepare an environment enriched with blood and nutrients to receive the fertilized egg. The fertilized egg then implants in this thickened uterine lining (endometrium). If the egg is not fertilized, it decays and is absorbed into the body, and the thickened uterine lining is expelled during menstruation.

EVALUATING INFERTILITY

Initial Evaluation

The cost of initial diagnostics range from a few hundred to several thousand dollars. The length of time, on average, to arrive at a diagnosis is 6 months for a woman and 1 month for a man (Patterson, 1991). The couple will be asked about childhood illnesses, injuries or surgeries, and any family infertility problems. Both partners' sexual histories are explored—whether either has had a sexually transmitted disease, previous pregnancies, or infections—as well as their current sexual habits, including whether the woman experiences pain during sex, a possible indication of infection or endometriosis (a condition in which the endometrium moves out of the uterus and attaches to the fallopian tubes or other areas of the reproductive tract). The physician will also inquire about the couple's lifestyle, asking questions about work, alcohol, nicotine, and other drug usage, exposure to toxic chemicals, and general stress level.

The woman's initial visit generally consists of the following: a review of her basal body temperature (BBT), her menstrual history (regularity, flow, cramps, etc.); a complete physical examination; a pelvic examination of the uterus, ovaries, and fallopian tubes; and lab analyses to determine whether there are any bacterial infections. Next, the physician usually suggests that the woman use an LH surge monitoring kit at home to determine when she is ovulating and to return when the test registers a surge. During her LH surge, the woman has blood taken at the physician's office to test her hormone levels. Other possible tests include a postcoital cervical mucus test and an ultrasound test.

Evaluation is much simpler for the male; the initial tests are completed during the first visit. The man has a complete physical examination, which may reveal signs of hormonal abnormalities. The physician examines the testicles and the rectum, then the man is asked to produce a sperm sample for analysis.

Advanced Evaluation

Prior to undergoing the following procedures, pregnancy tests are typically administered to insure that newly implanted embryos are not disturbed. A *hysterosalpingogram* (HSG) involves X-raying a woman whose reproductive tract has been injected with radiopaque dye. This test checks whether the fallopian tubes are open and whether there are any abnormalities in the reproductive tract. The HSG may reveal abnormalities in the shape of the uterus and any blockages, growths, polyps, or tumors in the fallopian tubes. Most women experience serious pain due to cramping during this procedure.

If abnormalities are detected during the HSG or an HSG is contraindicated, the physician may wish to perform a *hysteroscopy* to determine the presence of endometriosis and other pelvic adhesions. This procedure utilizes a *laparoscope;* a small incision is made just below the navel and a fiber optic laparoscope is inserted into the woman's abdominal cavity, which allows the physician to examine the outside of the reproductive organs. This procedure is not only diagnostic but can be used as a corrective procedure, as the doctor may proceed with a laparotomy to remove endometrial tissue or adhesions. Another exam, called an *endometrial biopsy* may be performed. It involves inserting a thin catheter into the uterus through the cervix and removing a small sample of the uterine lining to determine whether the hormonal levels are adequate to maintain implantation of the embryo.

Advanced evaluations for men include further analyses of the semen, examination of the sperm-producing tract, and hormonal testing. With an initial diagnosis of azoospermia (no sperm), several tests may be conducted including the fructose test, karotyping, or a testicular biopsy. Some men have a normal sperm profile yet are unable to fertilize an egg. Fertilizing capacity can be evaluated with the "hamster" test or sperm penetration assay (SPA or HPA). Men's semen should also be checked for these bacteria because sexual partners will be likely to share bacteria.

There may be several reasons for the absence of sperm in a man's ejaculate. He may have been born without a vas deferens—the tubes that connect his testicles to the ejaculatory duct where sperm mixes with semen; the sperm may be blocked from combining with his seminal fluid; the seminal fluid may not contain proper nourishment for the sperm; or, the man may not be producing any sperm at all. Sperm analysis should include the following: volume of the semen, sperm count, concentration per milliliter of semen, sperm motility (the percentage of sperm which are active), and sperm size and shape. Sperm count in fertile men ranges from 20–200 million sperm per milliliter and is not necessarily the most important measure of fertility. The physician will, for example, inquire about any urological surgery, pain, or other problems in the testicles; they will measure the testicles and feel their firmness, check whether the ducts that carry semen are present, and if there are any varicoceles (varicose veins in the scrotum). Only 15% of men have varicoceles, and not all of this group have impaired fertility. However, because varicose veins tend to worsen over time, varicoceles are present in 80% of men with secondary infertility.

TREATMENTS

Hormonal imbalances constitute a significant portion of infertility problems, particularly for women. Hormones are prescribed to treat a variety of problems in women including irregular ovulation, luteal phase defect (a hormonal imbalance that prevents implantation of the fertilized egg), endometriosis, and polycystic ovarian disease. Hormonal treatment can also be used as a possible way of preventing miscarriage once pregnancy has been achieved.

The following hormones are the most commonly used to regulate and increase ovulation: clomiphene citrate (CC; Clomid, Serophene), human menopausal gonadotropin (hMG; Pergonal, Humegon, and Metrodin); human chorionic gonadotropin (hCG; Profasi), gonadotropin-releasing hormone analogues (GnRH; Lupron). Hormones such as Lupron are routinely used in ART cycles to shut off the normal communication between the pituitary gland and the ovaries. This causes the lowering of estrogen levels to menopausal levels and gives physicians greater control over follicle stimulation so that a woman's menstrual cycle can coincide with that of her donor's. Other hormonal treatments include progesterone supplements, danocrine (Danazol), prednisone, dexamethasone, or spironolactone (Aldactone). In regard to usage of many of these hormonal treatments, there is relatively little research on repeated usage of these medications for treating infertility; possible problems are discussed below under the heading "Risks and Other Considerations."

Only about 5% of male factor infertility is due to hormonal problems (Marrs, 1997). Because men and women produce the same set of hormones at different levels, when required, men may be given the same hormonal treatments as women; however, the conditions they treat will be different.

Antibiotics may be one of the first protocols prescribed if bacterial infection has been discovered. It is particularly important to treat these infections before performing most surgical procedures on women because of the risk of introducing the bacteria into the upper reproductive tract. And, as mentioned above, it is essential to treat both partners so that one is not reinfected by the other.

Treatments for Women

Microsurgery is used in treating pelvic adhesions and endometriosis, reconstructing damaged sections of the reproductive tract, reversing sterilization, and removing tumors or cysts. Certain conditions such as endometriosis and pelvic adhesions can also be treated during laparoscopic surgery. Hysteroscopic surgery is used to treat certain uterine problems: uterine septum, intrauterine adhesions, polyps, or small fibroid tumors.

Treatments for Men

Most treatment for men involves surgery or *inseminations* with partner or donor sperm. Inseminations are relatively inexpensive, usually costing between $100 and $300, depending on whether the sperm is obtained from the partner or a donor. Inseminations are coordinated with the woman's ovulation, have a success rate of 20–25%, and, because a series of repeated cycles are usually suggested, treatment lasts for 6–8 months on average (Berger et al., 1995). Varicocelectomy for treatment of a varicocele is one of the most common surgeries for male factor infertility. Surgery is also undertaken to unblock ducts or vas deferens damaged from childhood hernia operations.

ASSISTED REPRODUCTIVE TECHNOLOGIES

If couples do not achieve a pregnancy using the above treatments, they may be candidates for ART. The *in vitro* fertilization (IVF) protocol is one in which folicle stimulating hormones such as Pergonal or Metrodin are used. The eggs that are produced are then surgically retrieved at ovulation, combined with the man's sperm in a petri dish, and incubated in the laboratory where they are fertilized and begin to divide. After 36–48 hours, the zygotes (fertilized egg cells) or preembryos are transferred by catheter into the woman's uterus, and, if one or more implant, pregnancy proceeds as normal.

Variations of IVF include gamete intrafallopian transfer (GIFT), in which sperm and eggs are combined and then reintroduced into a fallopian tube to fertilize; and zygote intrafallopian transfer (ZIFT), which is a combination of IVF and GIFT: fertilization occurs in a petri dish, and the zygotes are returned to the fallopian tube. Live birth rates for ART average approximately 23% for IVF, 27% for GIFT, and 28% for ZIFT per embryo transfer (SART, 1998). However, these rates decrease in relation to a woman's age; they dramatically drop to 6–7% after a woman reaches 40.

Previously irremediable male factor infertility now benefits from intracytoplasmic sperm injection (ICSI), a procedure in which the physician uses a microscopic needle to remove sperm from the testes and inject a single sperm directly into an egg. If fertilization is achieved, the procedure follows the standard IVF protocol. Recent data indicate that live birth rates with ICSI are comparable to or slightly higher than IVF performed without ICSI (SART, 1998).

Donors and Surrogates

When a partner cannot produce gametes, the next rung on the treatment ladder is the donation of either sperm or egg. On rare occasions, both are used. Egg donor procedures have higher live birth rates than standard IVF because donors are young and therefore produce more viable eggs. The success rate is 36% per embryo transfer (SART, 1998). This protocol is expensive, adding $3,000–$7,500 to the IVF cost.

When women are unable to carry a baby to term, some couples consider surrogacy. A surrogate is a woman who agrees to be inseminated with the husband's sperm (using her egg), to carry the baby to term, and to relinquish it to the couple at birth. Gestational surrogacy, a similar procedure, uses both partner's gametes, which are fertilized in vitro and then transferred to the uterus of the gestational carrier. Therefore, none of her genetic material is used. Surrogacy procedures are costly, with gestational surrogacy, which includes IVF, costing more.

RISKS AND OTHER CONSIDERATIONS

Clinicians need to be cognizant of the various side effects that hormonal treatments produce. These may include hot flashes, mood swings, breast tenderness, headaches, nervousness, dizziness, nausea and vomiting, weight gain, fatigue, and temporary visual disturbances (Marrs, 1997). Ovarian hyperstimulation syndrome, a condition in which the ovaries become swollen and painfully filled with cysts, may also result. Significant long-term effects for woman who have undergone 12 or more cycles may include an increased risk of ovarian tumors (Rossing et al., 1994).

Couples using ART have more than a 30% chance of having multiple births (SART, 1998). Multiple births place mothers and babies at greater health risk than single births. Multiples are often premature, with low birth weights, and are likely to have more health problems than babies delivered at term. When three or more embryos implant, physicians generally recommend what is called a *reduction*, a procedure in which the number of gestational sacs is reduced to improve the chances that the remaining fetuses will survive and be healthy infants. A dilemma posed by reduction is its potential to stimulate a spontaneous miscarriage of all the fetuses. In addition, reduction is essentially the same as a selective abortion and for that reason it may pose other problematic issues for some couples.

TABLE 1. Infertility: Causes, Evaluations, Treatments, Costs, and Success Rates

Common causes of infertility	Diagnostic tests	Treatment procedures	Costs per procedure	Success rates per procedure
Male factors 40%[a]				
Low sperm count	Semen analysis	Antibiotics	*	**
Poor sperm motility	Sperm penetration assay (hamster test)	Hormone treatment	*	**
Poor sperm morphology		ICSI (in combination with IVF)	$500–$2,500 (cost of IVF not included)	25% per embryo transfer[c]
		IUI	$150–300[a]	20–25%[b]
		DI	$225d	**
Varicocele	Physical examination Sonogram	Varicocelectomy	$1,500–$4,000[d]	50–60%[b]
Vasectomy	NA	Vasectomy reversal	$2,500–$6,000	**
Female factors 40%[a]				
Peritoneal factors (endometriosis)	Laparoscopy	Fertility medication	*	**
		Surgery	$2,500–$12,000	**
Ovulation factors	BBT chart	Fertility medication	$100–$2,000 per cycle	50%[b] 36%[c]
	LH surge kit Endometrial biopsy	Egg donor (in combination with IVF)	Cost for egg donor (without IVF) can vary from $3,000–$7,5000	
Tubal factors	Hysterosalpingogram	IVF	$8,000–$10,000	+
	Laparoscopy	GIFT–ZIFT	$8,000–$10,000	++
			$8,000–$10,000	30.5%[c]
Cervical factors	Postcoital test	Antibiotics	*	**
		Hormone treatment	*	**
		IUI	$150–$300[a]	20–25%[b]
Uterine factors	Hystero-salpingogram Hysteroscopy	Surgery	$3,000–$8,000	**
Interactive factors 10%[a]	Postcoital test	IUI	$150–$300[a]	20–25%[b]
Unexplained factors 10%[a]	All	Any and all		

Note. Structure of table derived from Meyers et al. (1995a).
[a]Marrs (1997); [b]Berger et al. (1995); [c]SART (1998); [d]Harkness (1992).
*Costs may vary; **Success rates not available.

+IVF success rates:
Women < 35 years with no male factor—27.5%
Women 35–39 years with no male factor—21.6%
Women > 39 with no male factor—10.6%
Women < 35 years with male factor—25.2%
Women 35–39 years with male factor—20.2%
Women > 39 years with male factor—6.6%

++GIFT success rates:
Women < 35 years with no male factor—36.4%
Women 35–39 years with no male factor—24.0%
Women > 39 years with no male factor—12.0%
Women < 35 years with male factor—32.9%
Women 35–39 years with male factor—33.7%
Women > 39 years with male factor—13.0%

REFERENCES

Abbey, A., Halman, L. J., & Andrews, F. M. (1992). Psychosocial, treatment, and demographic predictors of the stress associated with infertility. *Fertility and Sterility, 56,* 122–128.

Ackerman Institute for the Family's Infertility Project. (1995). *Couples and infertility: Moving beyond loss* [Video]. New York: Guilford Press.

Andrews, F. M., Abbey, A., & Halman, L. J. (1992). Is fertility-problem stress different? The dynamics of stress in fertile and infertile couples. *Fertility and Sterility, 57,* 1247–1253.

Baran, A., & Pannor, R. (1989). *Lethal secrets: The shocking consequences and unsolved problems of artificial insemination.* New York: Amistad/Warner Books.

Bartholet, E. (1993). *Family bonds: Adoption and the politics of parenting.* Boston: Houghton Mifflin.

Bassin, D. (1989). Women's shifting sense of self: The impact of reproductive technology. In J. Offerman-Zuckerberg (Ed.), *Gender in transition* (pp. 189–202). New York: Plenum.

Becker, G. (1990). *Healing the infertile family: Strengthening your relationship in the search for parenthood.* New York: Bantam Books.

Belsky, J., & Rovine, M. (1990). Patterns of marital change across the transition to parenthood: Pregnancy to three years postpartum. *Journal of Marriage and the Family, 52,* 5–19.

Benedek, T. (1952). Infertility as a psychosomatic defense. *Fertility and Sterility, 3,* 527–541.

Berg, B. J., & Wilson, J. F. (1991). Psychological functioning across stages of treatment for infertility. *Journal of Behavioral Medicine, 14,* 11–26.

Berg, B. J., Wilson, J. F., & Weingartner, P. L. (1991). Psychological sequelae of

231

infertility treatment: The role of gender and sex-role identification. *Society, Science, and Medicine, 33*, 1071–1080.

Berger, G. S., Goldstein, M., & Fuerst, M. (1995). *The couple's guide to infertility: Updated with the newest scientific techniques to help you have a baby* (rev. ed.). New York: Main Street Books/Doubleday.

Bernstein, J., Mattonx, J. H., & Kellner, R. (1988). Psychological status of previously infertile couples after a successful pregnancy. *Journal of Gynecological and Neonatal Nursing, 17*, 404–408.

Boivan, J., Takefman, J., Tulandi, T., & Brender, W. (1995). Reactions to infertility based on extent of treatment failure. *Fertility and Sterility, 63*, 801–807.

Bombardieri, M. (1983, December 5). The twenty-minute talk rule: First aid for couples in distress. *Resolve Newsletter*. Somerville, MA: RESOLVE.

Boss, P. (1991). Ambiguous loss. In F. Walsh & M. McGoldrick (Eds.), *Living beyond loss: Death in the family* (pp. 164–175). New York: Norton.

Bowen, M. (1976). Theory in the practice of psychotherapy. In P. Guerin (Ed.), *Family therapy: Theory and practice* (pp. 42–91). New York: Gardner Press.

Braverman, A., & Corson, S. (1995). Factors related to preferences in gamete donor sources. *Fertility and Sterility, 63*, 543–549.

Brinich, P. M. (1990). Adoption from the inside out: A psychoanalytic perspective. In D. Brodzinsky & M. Schechter (Eds.), *The psychology of adoption* (pp. 42–46). New York: Oxford University Press.

Brodzinsky, D. M., Schechter, M. D., & Henig, R. M. (1992). *Being adopted: The lifelong search for self*. New York: Doubleday.

Burns, L. H. (1990). An exploratory study of perceptions of parenting after infertility. *Family Systems Medicine, 8*, 177–189.

Carter, B., & McGoldrick, M. (1989). Overview. In B. Carter & M. McGoldrick (Eds.), *The changing family life cycle* (2nd ed., pp. 3–28). Boston: Allyn & Bacon.

Carter, J. W., & Carter, M. (1989). *Sweet grapes: How to stop being infertile and start living again*. Indianapolis, IN: Perspectives Press.

Clamar, A. (1980). Psychological implications of donor insemination. *American Journal of Psychoanalysis, 40*, 173–177.

Collins, A., Freeman, E. W., Boxer, A. S., & Tureck, R. (1992). Perceptions of infertility and treatment stress in females as compared with males entering in vitro fertilization treatment. *Fertility and Sterility, 57*, 350–356.

Daniluk, J. C. (1988). Infertility: Intrapersonal and interpersonal impact. *Fertility and Sterility, 49*, 982–990.

Diamond, R. (1995). Secrecy vs. privacy. *Adoptive Families, 28*, 8–11.

Domar, A., Seibel, M., & Benson, H. (1990). The mind/body program for infertility: A new behavioral treatment approach for women with infertility. *Fertility and Sterility, 53*, 246–249.

Eisner, B. G. (1963). Some psychological differences between fertile and infertile women. *Journal of Clinical Psychology, 19*, 391–394.

Faludi, S. (1991). *Backlash: The undeclared war against American women*. New York: Crown.

Fein, E. (1998, January 25). For lost pregnancies, new rites of mourning. *The New York Times*, pp. A1, A34.

Fertility for sale. (1998, March 5). *The New York Times*, p. A21.

Freeman, E. W., Boxer, A. S., Rickels, K., Tureck, R., & Mastrioanni, L. (1985). Psychological evaluation and support in a program of in vitro fertilization and embryo transfer. *Fertility and Sterility, 43,* 48–53.

Golombok, S., Cook, R., Bish, A., & Murray, C. (1995). Families created by the new reproductive technologies: Quality of parenting and social and emotional development of the children. *Child Development, 66,* 285–298.

Gonzalez, S., Steinglass, P., & Reiss, D. (1989). Putting the illness in its place: Discussion groups for families with chronic illnesses. *Family Process, 28,* 69–87.

Gordon, E. R. (1992). *Mommy, did I grow in your tummy?* Santa Monica, CA: E. M. Greenberg Press.

Greenfeld, D. A. (1995, October). *Children of IVF: What their parents have to say.* Paper presented at the 51st annual meeting of the American Society for Reproductive Medicine, Seattle, WA.

Greil, A. L. (1991). *Not yet pregnant.* New Brunswick, NJ: Rutgers University Press.

Grotevant, H. D., & McRoy, R. G. (1990). Adopted adolescents in residential treatment: The role of the family. In D. Brodzinsky & M. Schechter (Eds.), *The psychology of adoption* (pp. 167–186). New York: Oxford University Press.

Harbour, F. H. (1997, November–December). The new fertility. *Harvard Magazine,* pp. 54–99.

Harkness, C. (1992). *The infertility book: A comprehensive medical and emotional guide.* Berkeley, CA: Celestial Arts.

Hartman, A. (1993). Secrecy in adoption. In E. Imber-Black (Ed.), *Secrets in families and family therapy* (pp. 91–95). New York: Norton.

Hendricks, M. C. (1985). Feminist therapy with women and couples who are infertile. In L. B. Rosewater & L. E. A. Walker (Eds.), *Handbook of feminist therapy: Women's issues in psychotherapy* (pp. 147–158). New York: Springer.

Hirsch, A. M., & Hirsch, S. M. (1989). The effect of infertility on marriage and self-concept. *Journal of Obstetric, Gynecologic, and Neonatal Nursing, 18,* 13–20.

Humphrey, M. (1986). Infertility as a marital crisis. *Stress Medicine, 2,* 221–224.

Imber-Black, E. (Ed.). (1993). *Secrets in families and family therapy.* New York: Norton.

Imber-Black, E., & Roberts, J. (1993). *Rituals for our times: Celebrating, healing, and changing our lives and our relationships.* New York: HarperPerennial.

Ireland, M. (1993). *Reconceiving women.* New York: Guilford Press.

Johnson, P. E. (1994). *Taking charge of infertility.* Indianapolis, IN: Perspectives Press.

Jones, H. W., Jr., & Toner, J. P. (1993). The infertile couple. *New England Journal of Medicine, 329,* 1710–1715.

Karpel, M. A. (1980). Family secrets: I. Conceptual and ethical issues in the relational context. II. Ethical and practical considerations in therapeutic management. *Family Process, 19,* 295–306.

Kedem, P., Mikulincer, M., Nathanson, Y. E., & Bartov, B. (1990). Psychological aspects of male infertility. *British Journal of Medical Psychology, 63,* 73–80.

Kirkley-Best, E., & Kellner, K. (1982). The forgotten grief: A review of the psychology of stillbirth. *American Journal of Orthopsychiatry, 52,* 420–429.

Kolata, G. (1998, February 25). Price soars for eggs, setting off a debate on a clinic's ethics. *The New York Times,* pp. A1, A16.

Kraft, A., Palumbo, J., Mitchell, D., Dean, C., Meyers, S., & Schmitt, A. W. (1980). The psychological dimensions of infertility. *American Journal of Orthopsychiatry, 50,* 618–628.

Lalos, A., Lalos, O., Jacobsson, L., & Von Schultz, B. (1985). The psychosocial impact of infertility 2 years after completed surgical treatment. *Acta Obstetrica et Gynecologica Scandinavica, 64,* 599–604.

Lieber Wilkins, C. M. (1995, October). *Talking to children about their conception: A parent's perspective.* Paper presented at the 51st annual meeting of the American Society for Reproductive Medicine, Seattle, WA.

Lifton, B. J. (1998, February). *The secret life of the adopted child.* Paper presented at the 22nd annual scientific conference sponsored by the Washington Square Institute and the National Association of Adoption Counselors, New York.

Litt, M. D., Tennen, H., Affleck, G., & Klock, S. (1992). Coping and cognitive factors in adaptation to in vitro fertilization failure. *Journal of Behavioral Medicine, 15,* 171–187.

Mahlstedt, P. P. (1985). Psychological components of infertility. *Fertility and Sterility, 43,* 335–346.

Marrs, R. (with Bloch, L. F., & Silverman, K. K.). (1997). *Dr. Richard Marrs' fertility book.* New York: Delacorte Press.

Mathews, R. (1991, November). *The value and meaning of children for infertile couples.* Paper presented at the meeting of the National Council on Family Relations, Denver, CO.

Mathews, R., & Mathews, A. M. (1986). Infertility and involuntary childlessness: The transition to non-parenthood. *Journal of Marriage and the Family, 48,* 641–649.

Mathews, R., & Mathews, A. M. (1993, March). *Confronting infertility: Differences between men and women in accepting infertility and seeking medical treatment.* Paper presented in the Social Medicine Seminar Series, Department of Public Health and Care, University of Oxford, UK.

McDaniel, S. H., Hepworth, J., & Doherty, W. (1992). Medical family therapy with couples facing infertility. *American Journal of Family Therapy, 20,* 101–122.

McEwan, K. L., Costello, C. G., & Taylor, P. J. (1987). Adjustment to infertility. *Journal of Abnormal Psychology, 96,* 108–116.

McGoldrick, M., & Gerson, R. (1985). *Genograms and family assessment.* New York: Norton.

Melina, L. R. (1989). *Making sense of adoption: A parent's guide.* New York: Harper & Row.

Menning, B. E. (1988). *Infertility: A guide for the childless couple* (2nd ed.). New York: Prentice Hall Press.

Merck Manual (16th ed.). (1992). Philadelphia: National.

Meyers, M., Diamond, R., Kezur, D., Scharf, C., Weinshel, M., & Rait, D. S. (1995a). An infertility primer for family therapists: I. Medical, social, and psychological dimensions. *Family Process, 34,* 219–229.

Meyers, M., Diamond, R., Kezur, D., Scharf, C., Weinshel, M., & Rait, D. S. (1995b). An infertility primer for family therapists: II. Working with couples who struggle with infertility. *Family Process, 34,* 231–240.

Miall, C. E. (1987). The stigma of adoptive parent status: Perceptions of community attitudes toward adoption and the experience of informal social sanctioning. *Family Relations, 36,* 34–39.

Morse, C., & Dennerstein, L. (1985). Infertile couples entering an in vitro fertilization program: A preliminary survey. *Journal of Psychosomatic Obstetrics and Gynaecology, 4,* 207–219.

Mosher, W. D., & Pratt, W. F. (1990). *Fecundity and infertility in the United States 1965–1988: 192.* Washington, DC: National Center for Health Statistics.

Myers, M. (1990). Male gender-related issues in reproduction and technology. In N. L. Stotland (Ed.), *Psychiatric aspects of reproductive technology* (pp. 25–34). Washington, DC: American Psychiatric Press.

Nachtigall, R. D., Becker, G., & Wozny, M. (1992). The effects of gender specific diagnosis on men's and women's response to infertility. *Fertility and Sterility, 57,* 113–121.

New York State Task Force on Life and the Law. (1998). *Assisted reproductive technologies: Analysis and recommendations for public policy* (pp. 235–288). New York: Author.

O'Moore, A. M., O'Moore, R. R., Harrison, R. F., & Carruthers, M. (1983). Psychosomatic aspects in idiopathic infertility: Effects of treatment with autogenic training. *Journal of Psychosomatic Research, 27,* 145–151.

Olivennes, F., Derbrat, V., Rufat, P., Blanchet, V., Fanchin, R., & Frydman, R. (1997). Follow-up of a cohort of 422 children aged 6 to 13 years conceived by in vitro fertilization. *Fertility and Sterility, 67,* 284–289.

Orenstein, P. (1995, June 18). Looking for a donor to call Dad. *The New York Times Magazine,* pp. 28–35, 42, 50.

Patterson, J. (1991, October). *Systems therapy for infertile couples.* Paper presented at the annual meeting of the American Association for Marriage and Family Therapy, Washington, DC.

Penn, P. (1985). Feed-forward: Future questions, future maps. *Family Process, 24,* 299–310.

Peoples, D., & Ferguson, H. R. (1998). *Experiencing infertility.* New York: Norton.

Rolland, J. S. (1994). In sickness and in health: The impact of illness on couple's relationships. *Journal of Marital and Family Therapy, 20,* 327–347.

Rossing, M. A., Daling, J. R., Weiss, N. S., Moore, D. E., & Self, S. G. (1994). Ovarian tumors in a cohort of infertile women. *New England Journal of Medicine, 331,* 771–776.

Salzer, L. (1996, March). *Parenting after infertility.* Paper presented at the Spence Chapin Adoption Resource Center, New York.

Sandelowski, M. (1993). *With child in mind.* Philadelphia: University of Pennsylvania Press.

Sandelowski, M., & Jones, L. C. (1986). Social exchanges of infertile women. *Issues in Mental Health Nursing, 8,* 173–189.

SART. (1998). Assisted reproductive technology in the United States and Canada: 1995 results generated from the American Society for Reproductive Medicine/Society for Assisted Reproductive Technology Registry. *Fertility and Sterility, 69,* 389–396.

Schaffer, J., & Diamond, R. (1993). Infertility: Private pain and secret stigma. In E. Imber-Black (Ed.), *Secrets in families and family therapy* (pp. 106–120). New York: Norton.

Scharf, C., & Weinshel, M. (in press). Infertility and late life pregnancy. In P. Papp (Ed.), *Couples on the fault line: Contemporary couples therapy.* New York: Guilford Press.

Seibel, M., & Taymor, M. (1982). Emotional aspects of infertility. *Fertility and Sterility, 37,* 137–145.

Shapiro, S. (1988). Psychological consequences of infertility. In J. J. Offerman-Zuckerberg (Ed.), *Critical psychosocial passages in the life of a woman: A psychoanalytic perspective* (pp. 269–289). New York: Plenum Medical.

Shaw, P., Johnston, M., & Shaw, R. (1988). Counselling needs, emotional and relationship problems in couples awaiting IVF. Psychosocial and ethical concerns in new reproductive technologies. *Journal of Psychosomatic Obstetrics and Gynaecology* [Special issue], *9,* 171–180.

Simons, H. F. (1995). *Wanting another child: Coping with secondary infertility.* New York: Lexington Books.

Sorosky, A. D. (1995, October). *Lessons from the adoption experience: Anticipating times of developmental conflict for the ART child.* Paper presented at the 51st annual meeting of the American Society for Reproductive Medicine, Seattle, WA.

Tomm, K. (1987a). Interventive interviewing: Part I. Strategizing as a fourth guideline for the therapist. *Family Process, 26,* 3–13.

Tomm, K. (1987b). Interventive interviewing: Part II. Reflexive questioning as a means to enable self-healing. *Family Process, 26,* 167–183.

Tomm, K. (1987c). Interventive interviewing: Part III. Intending to ask lineal, circular, strategic, or reflexive questions? *Family Process, 27,* 1–15.

U.S. Office of Technology Assessment. (1988). *Infertility: Medical and social choices* (Publication No. OTA-BA-358). Washington, DC: U.S. Government Printing Office.

Ulbrich, P. M., Tremaglio-Coyle, A., & Llabre, M. M. (1990). Involuntary childlessness and marital adjustment: His and hers. *Journal of Sex and Marital Therapy, 16,* 147–158.

Veevers, J. E. (1980). *Childless by choice.* Toronto: Butterworth.

Walter, H. (1982). Psychological and legal aspects of artificial insemination (AID): An overview. *American Journal of Psychotherapy, 36,* 91–102.

Watkins, M., & Fisher, S. (1993). *Talking with young children about adoption.* New Haven, CT: Yale University Press.

White, M. (1989). *The externalizing of the problem and the re-authoring of lives and relationships: Selected papers.* Adelaide, Australia: Dulwich Centre.

White, M., & Epston, D. (1990). *Narrative means to therapeutic ends.* New York: Norton.

Whittemore, A. S. (1994). The risk of ovarian cancer after treatment for infertility. *New England Journal of Medicine, 331,* 805–806.

Wirtberg, I. (1992). *His and her childlessness.* Doctoral dissertation in Medical Science, Karolinska Institutet, Stockholm, Sweden.

Wright, J., Bissonnette, F., Duchesne, C., Benoit, J., Sabourin, S., & Girard, Y. (1991). Psychosocial distress and infertility: Men and women respond differently. *Fertility and Sterility, 55,* 100–108.

Zolbrod, A. P. (1993). *Men, women, and infertility.* New York: Lexington Books.

INDEX